I0163140

1

To study and sometimes

practice what one has learned,

is this not a pleasure?

— CONFUCIUS

Eight Pieces of Brocade – A Signs of Learning® Book
   The All-My-Life Exercise
   for Children Young & Old

Dedicated to Professor Huo Chi-Kwang (1896–1988),
who founded the Chinese Cultural Academy in 1966.

In appreciation to his former student, Master Louis A. Ucha,
Tai Chi Chuan teacher, Evanston, Illinois

Title: Murray David Harwich, Jr.

Registered Title: Murray David Harwich III

Text ©2017 Mary Belle Harwich

Paintings ©2017 Peggy Macnamara

Drawings ©2017 Charlotte Hart

End Quote: Lewis Carroll

ALL RIGHTS RESERVED

Printed in the United States

Published Frankfort, KY

Book Designs by Marjorie Snelson Design

ISBN 978-0-9888972-8-1

Library of Congress Control Number: 2019913507

To order printed books: www.amazon.com

Eight Pieces of Brocade
The All•My•Life Exercise
For Children Young & Old

A Signs of Learning Ü Book

Text – Mary Belle Harwich

Paintings – Peggy Macnamara

Drawings – Charlotte Hart

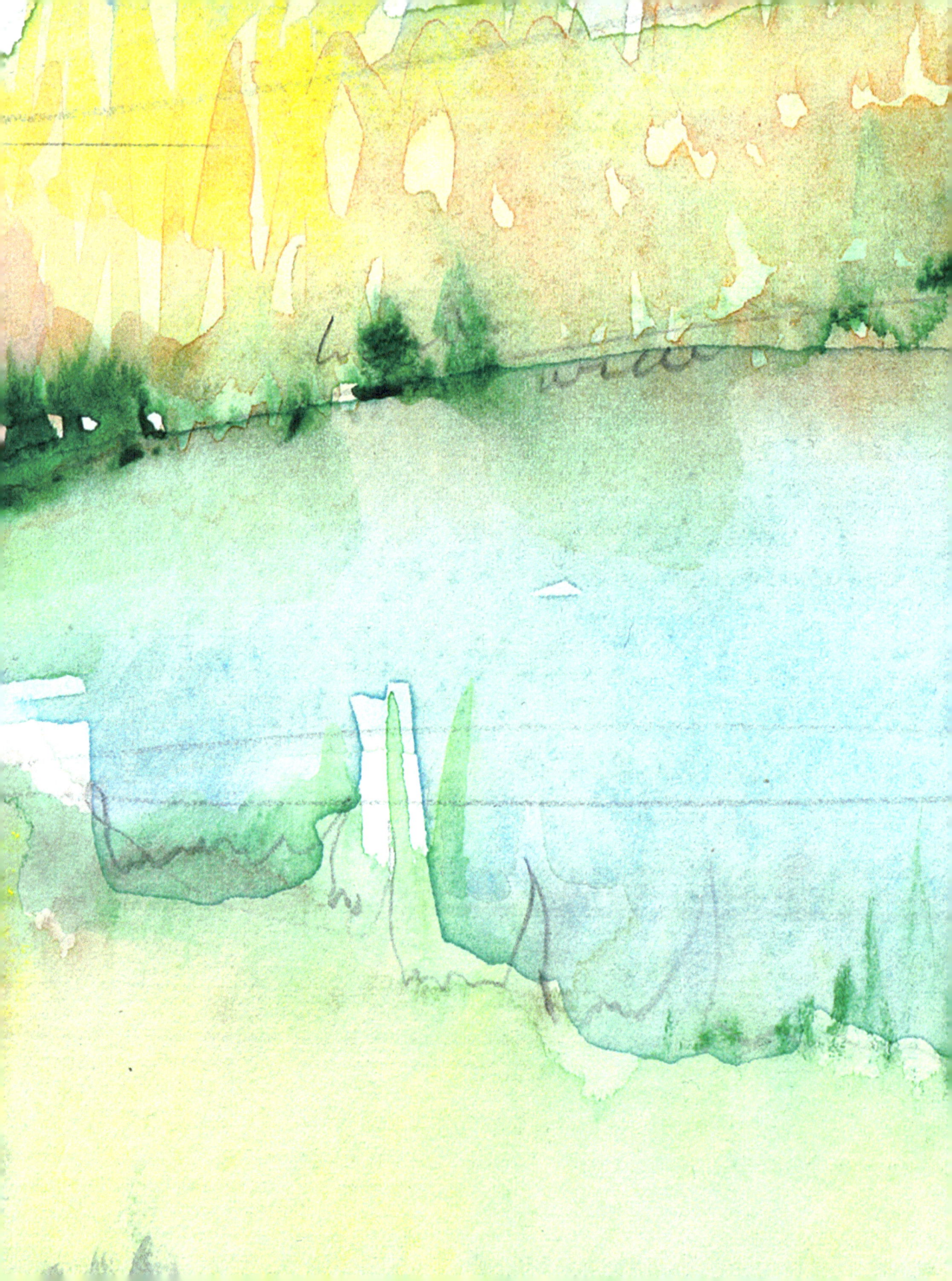

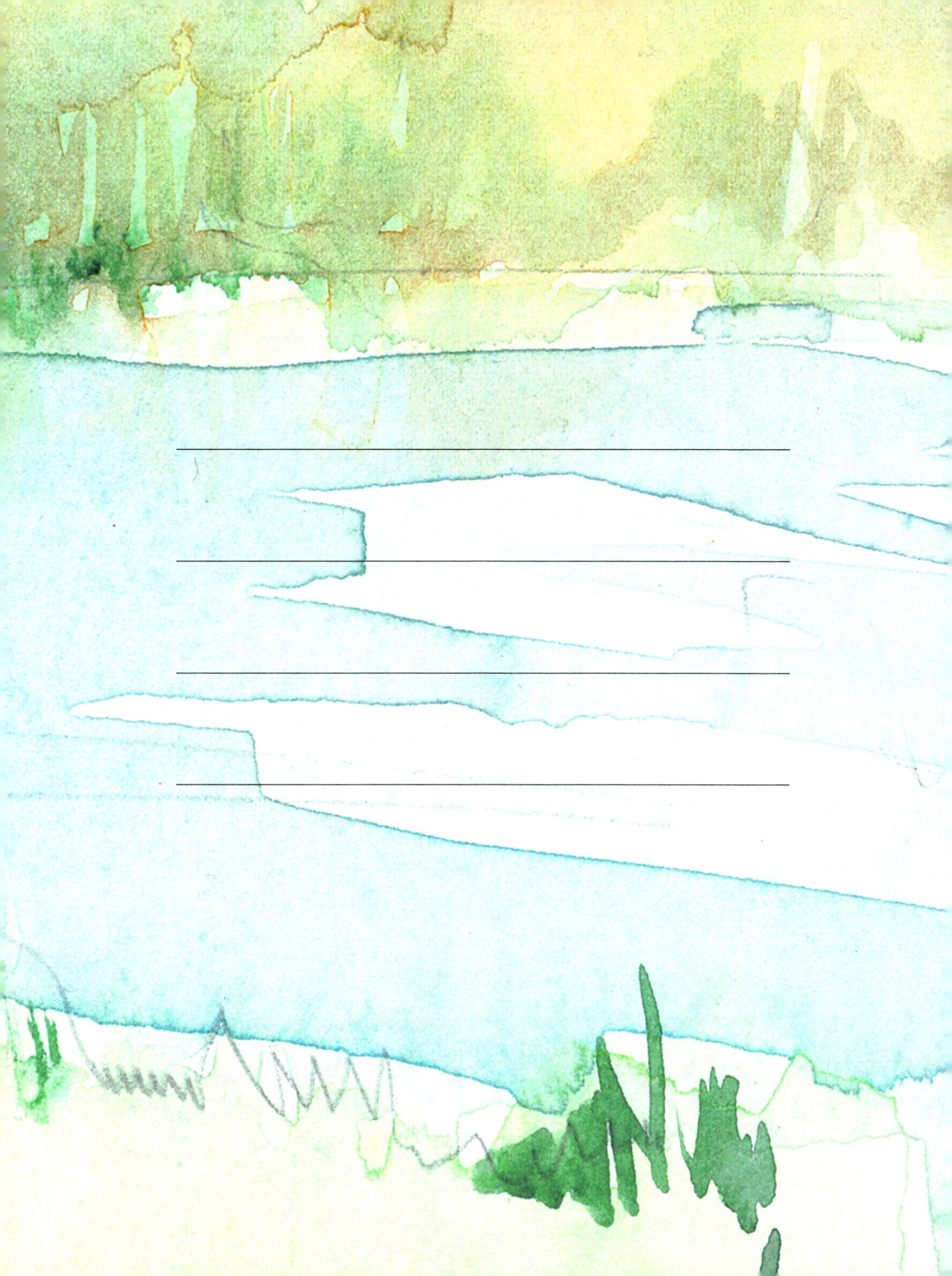

Do You Know?

Have You Heard?

Practice Is...

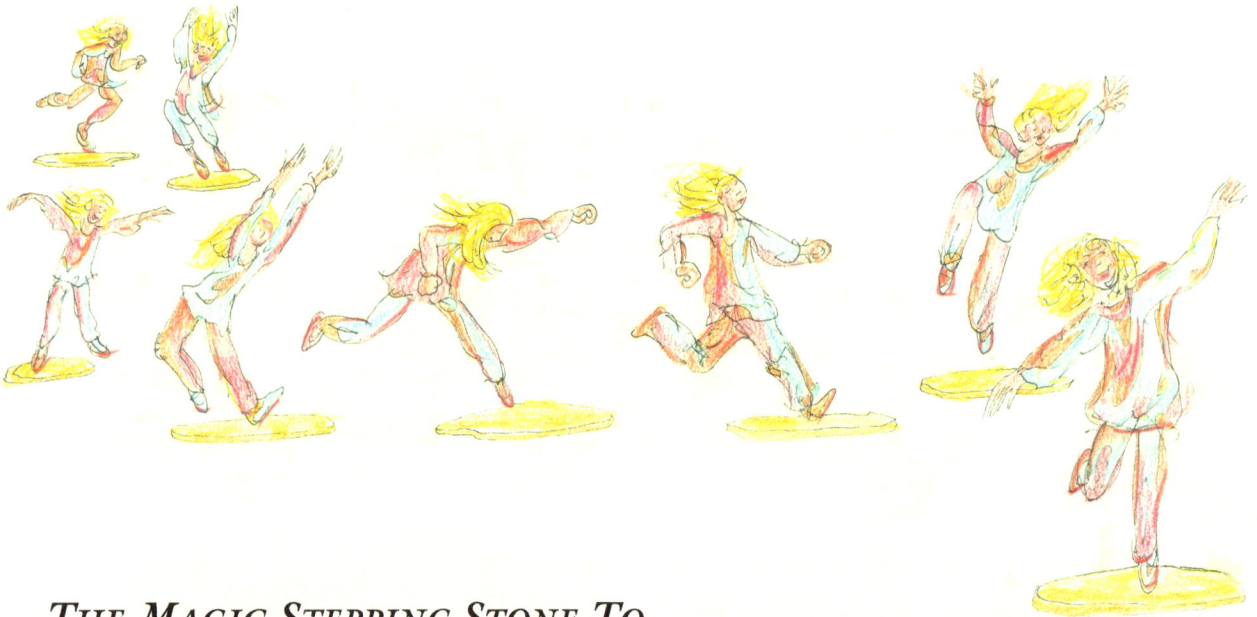

The Magic Stepping Stone To

Strength and Balance...

Practice once or many times...

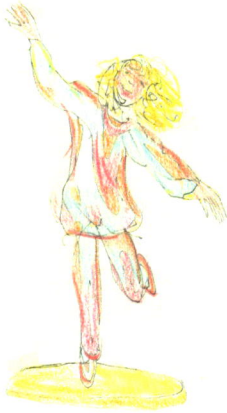

standing...

sitting...

or lying down...

back and forth...

or walking around...

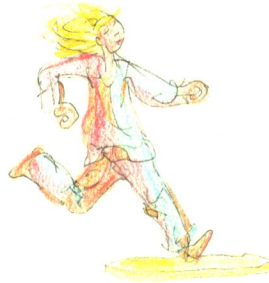

Let's begin...

White Crane spreads its wings…

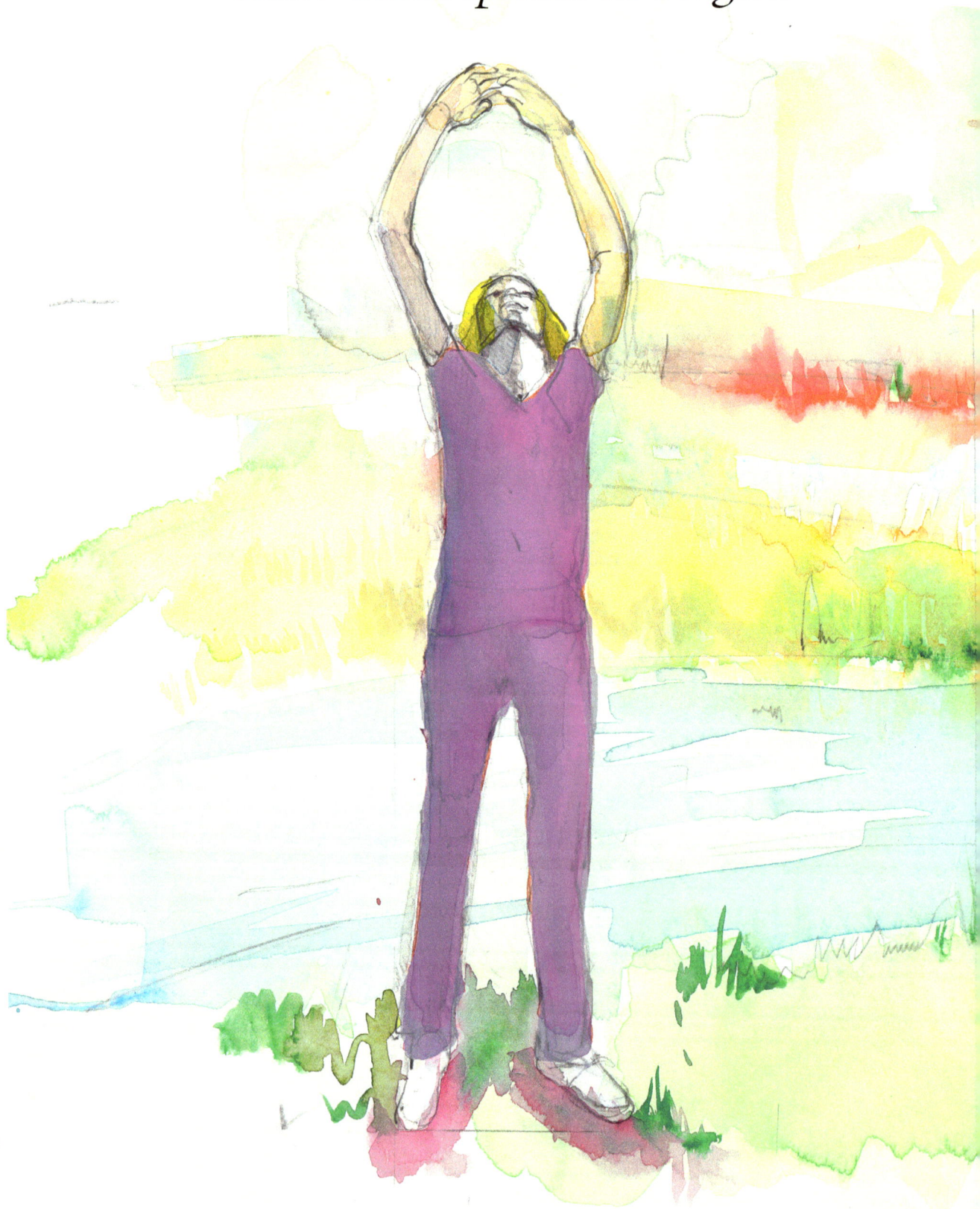

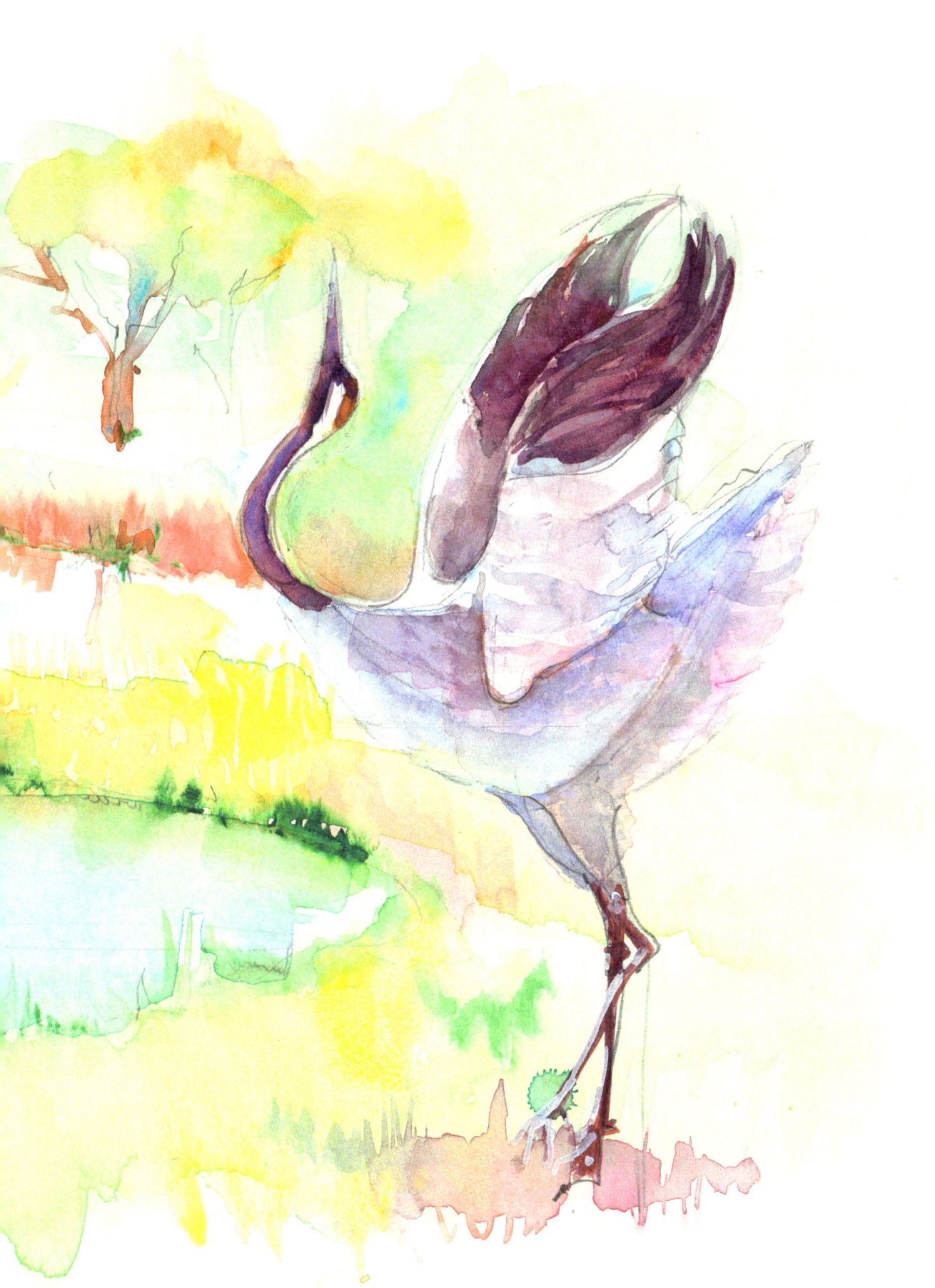

Smiling Sloth reaches out…

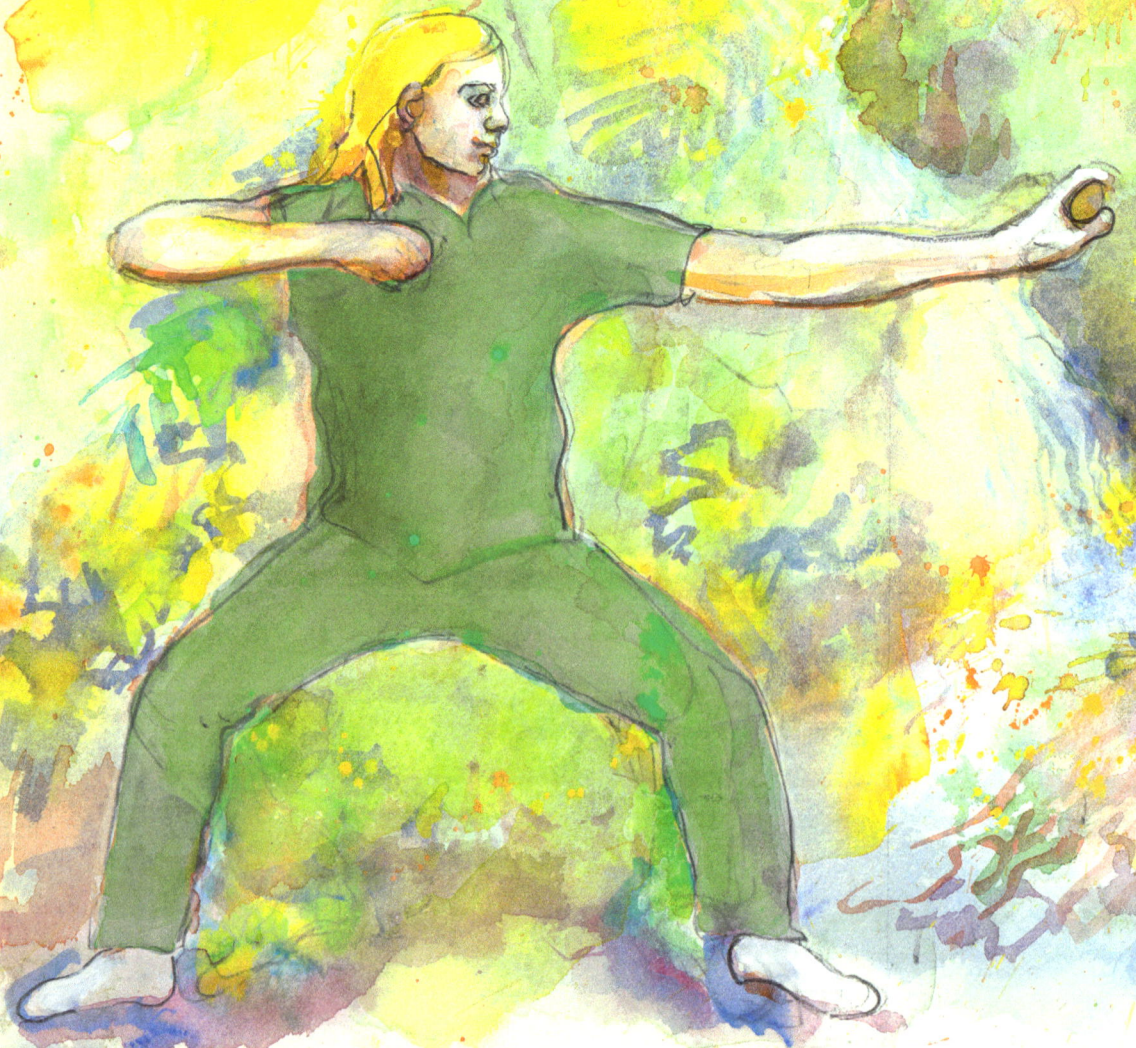

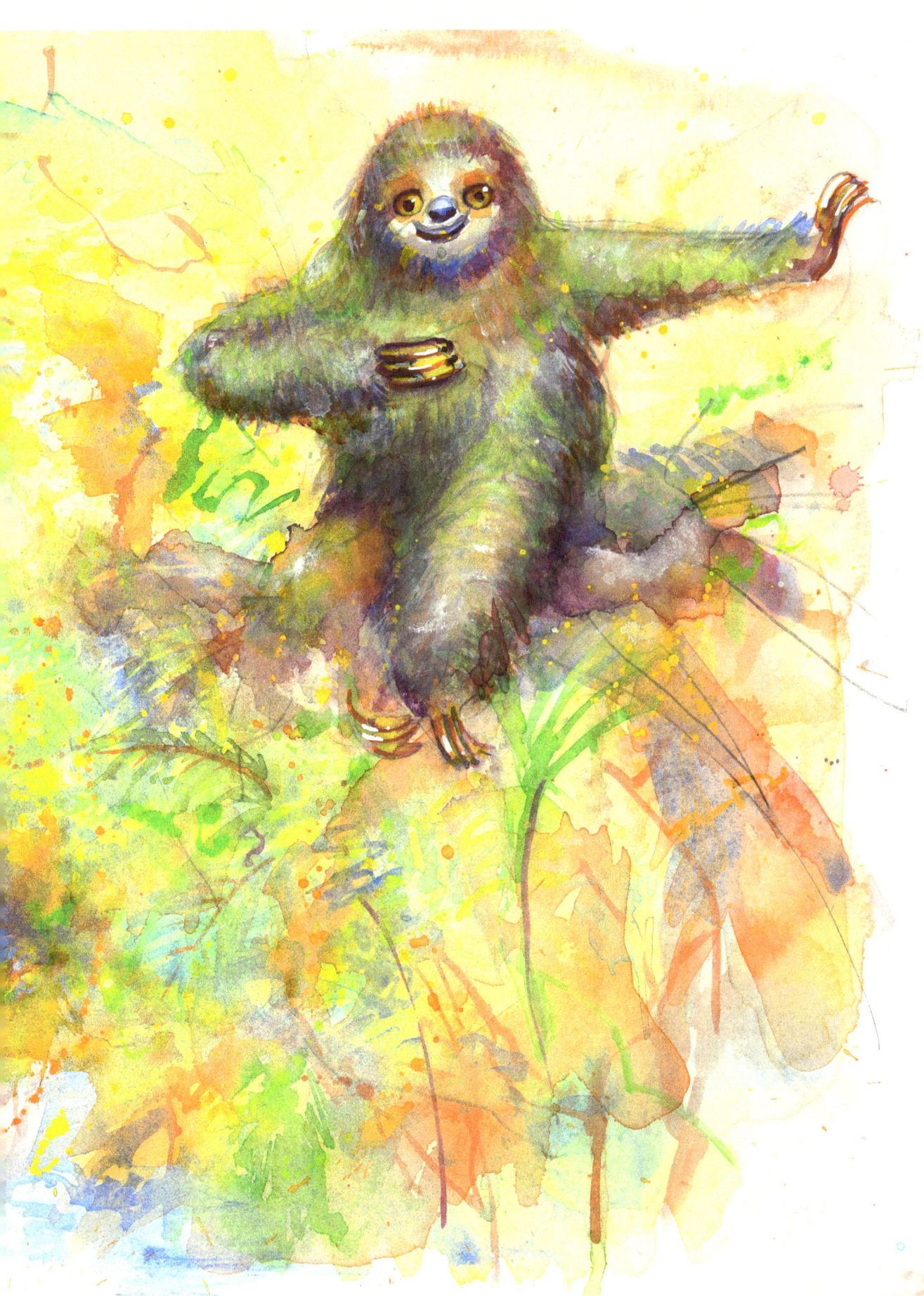

Nimble Monkey hangs on the branch...

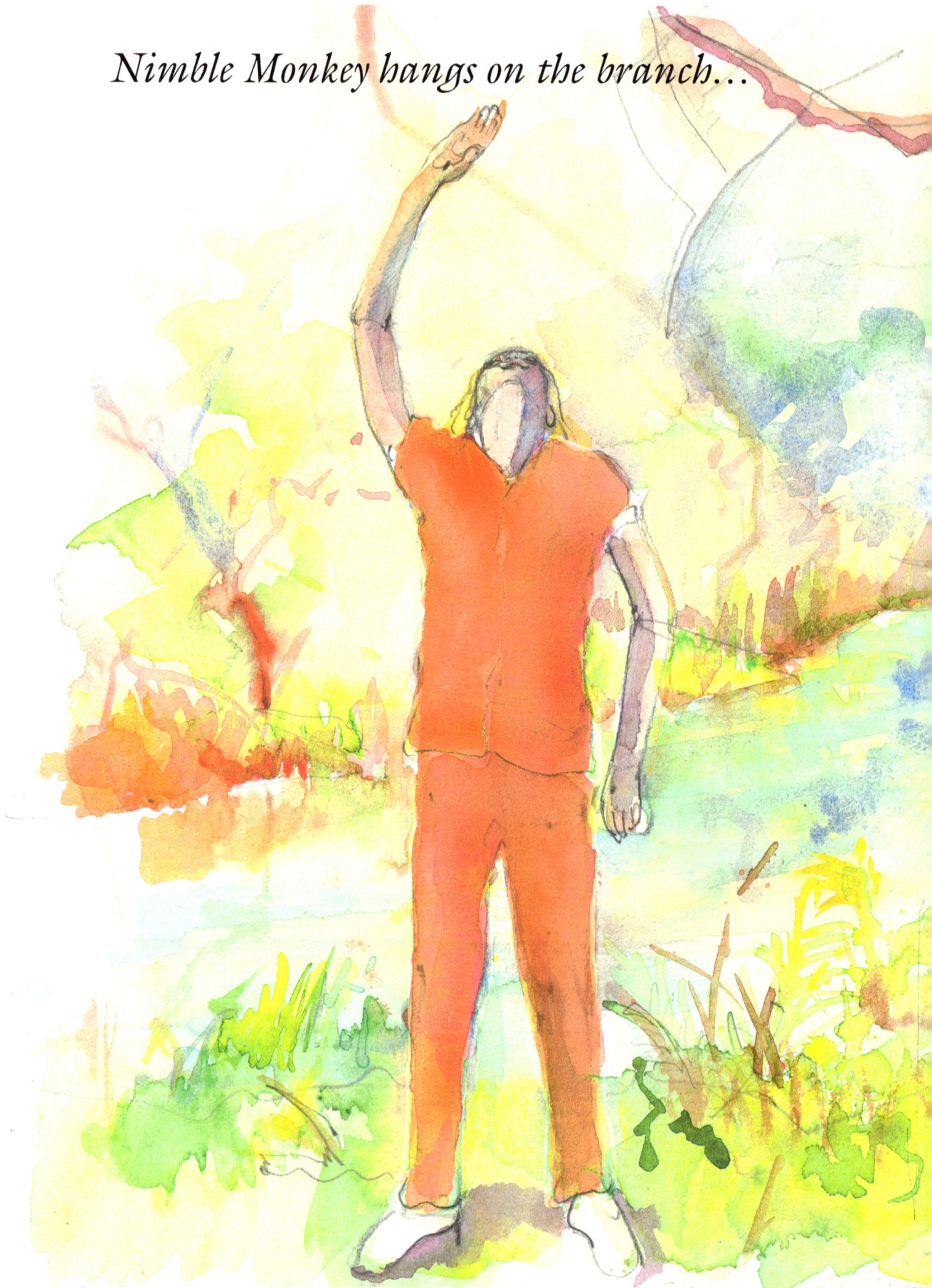

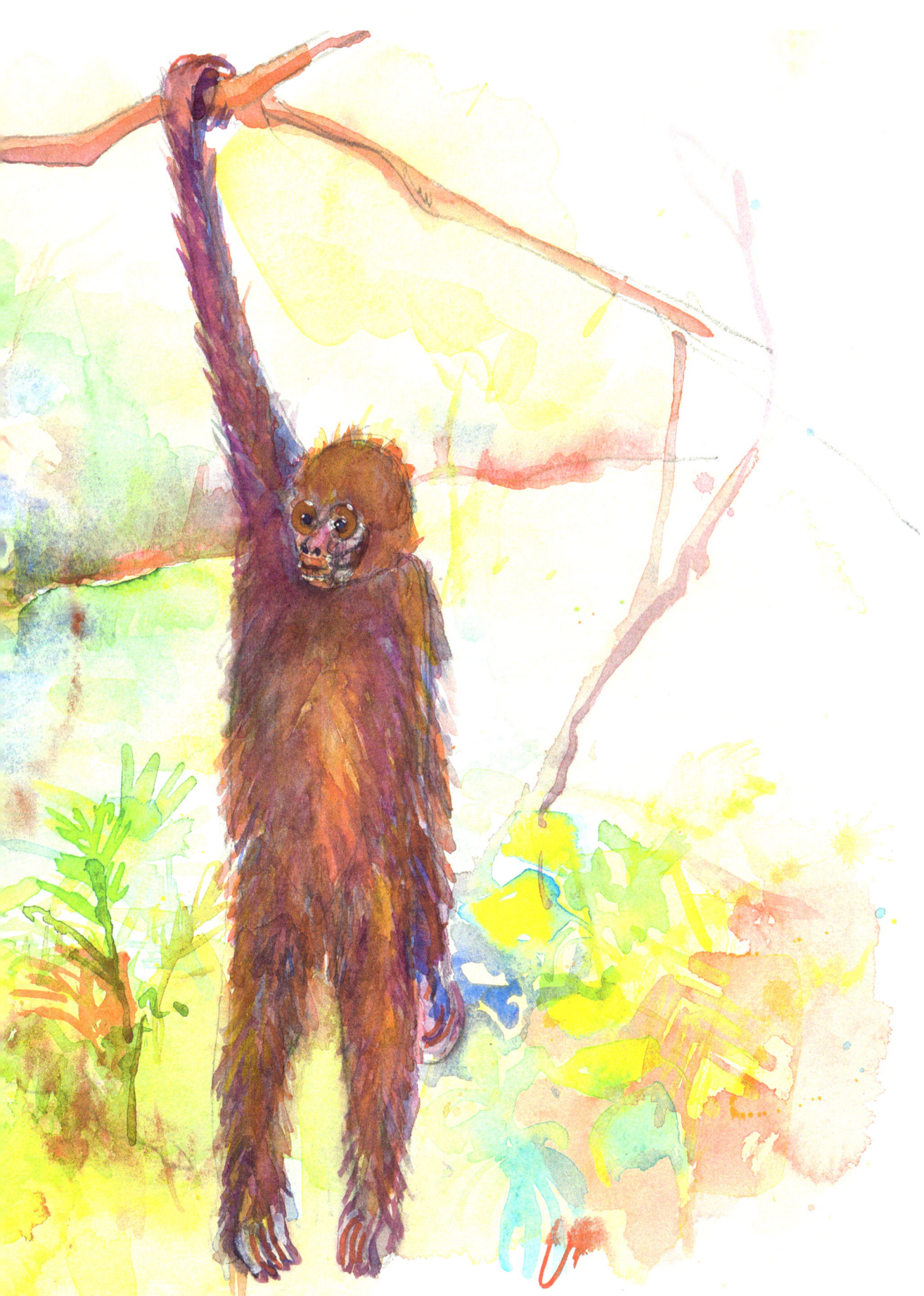

Wise Owl looks back – right then left...

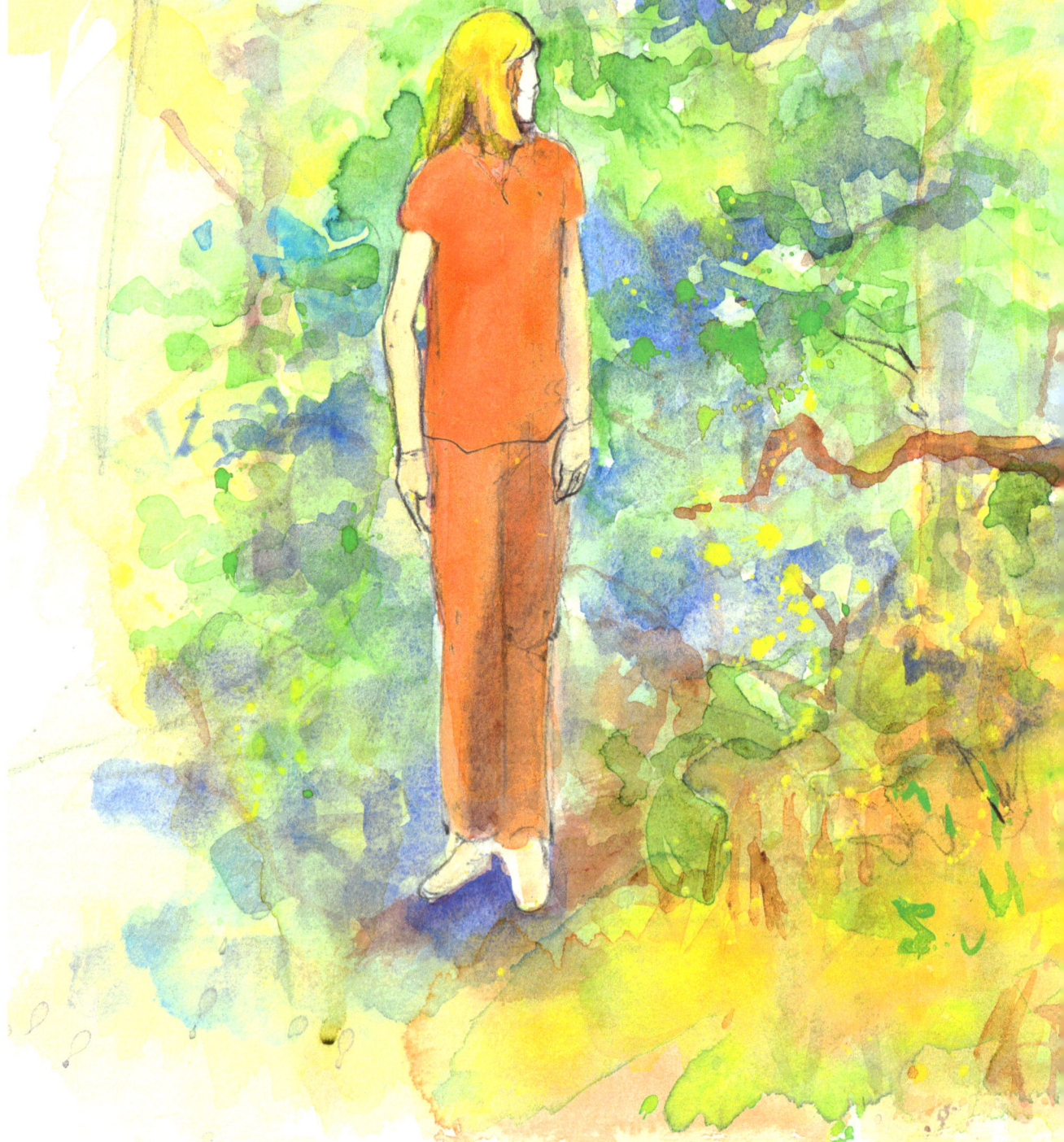

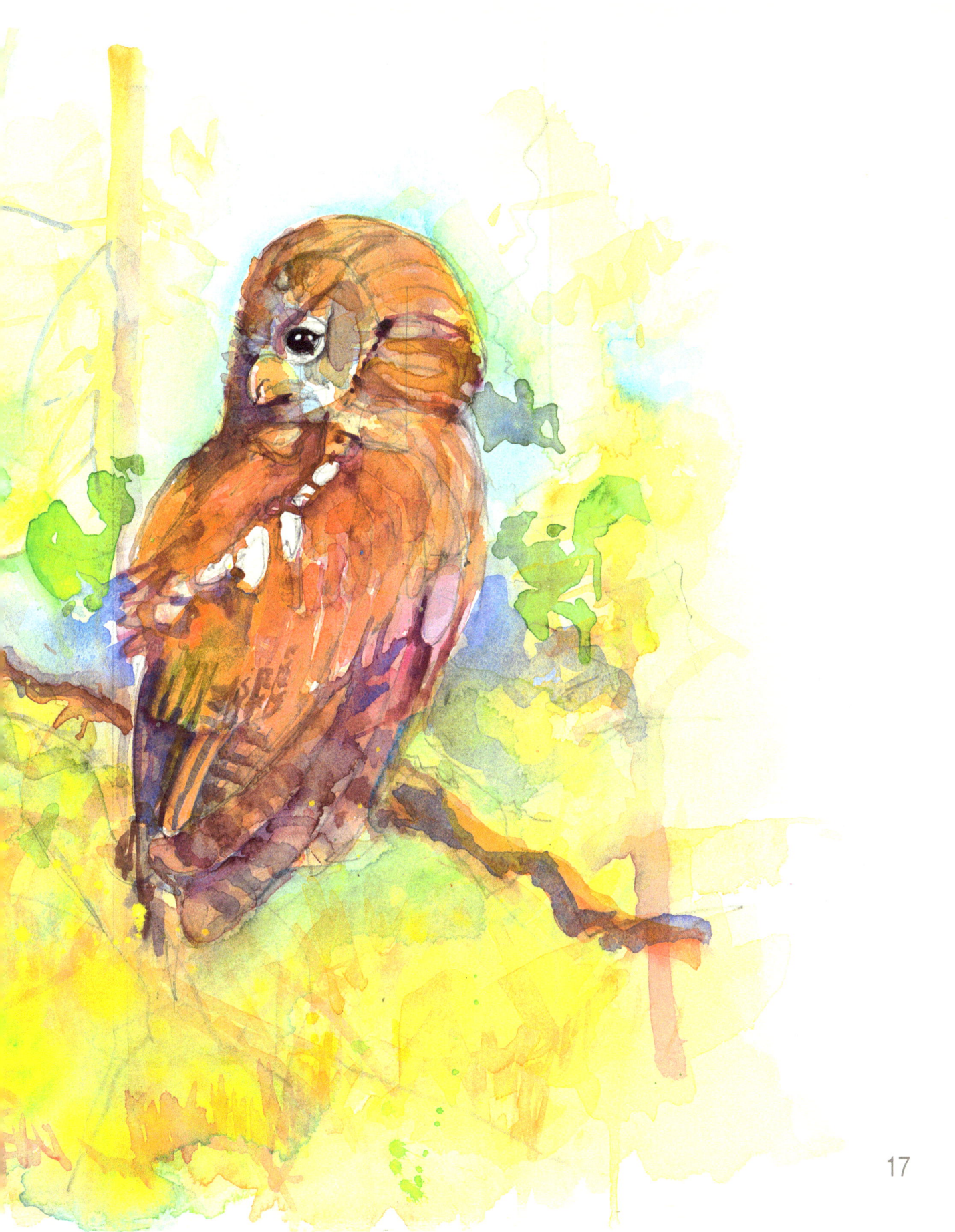

Crouching Cat sways side to side...

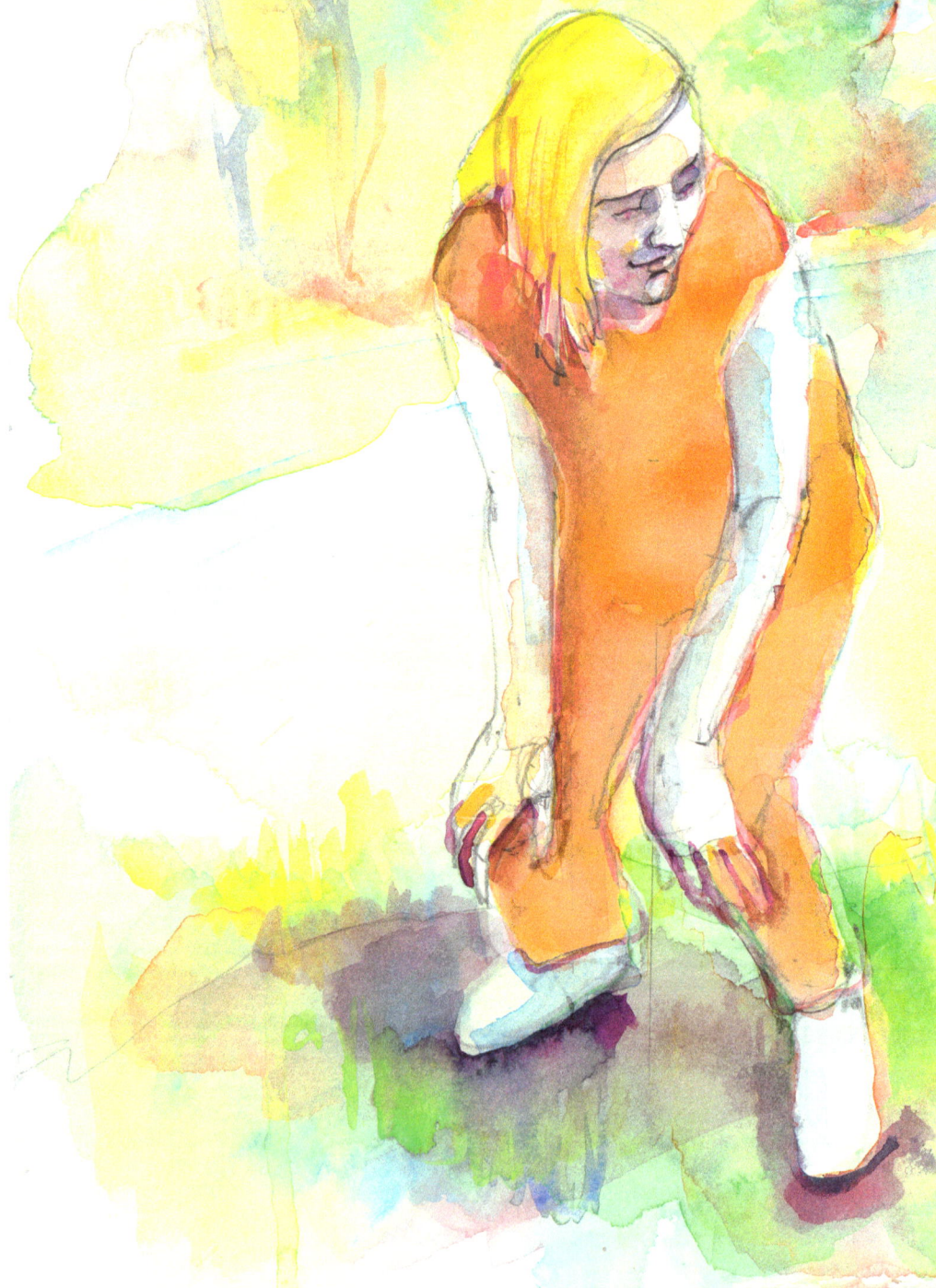

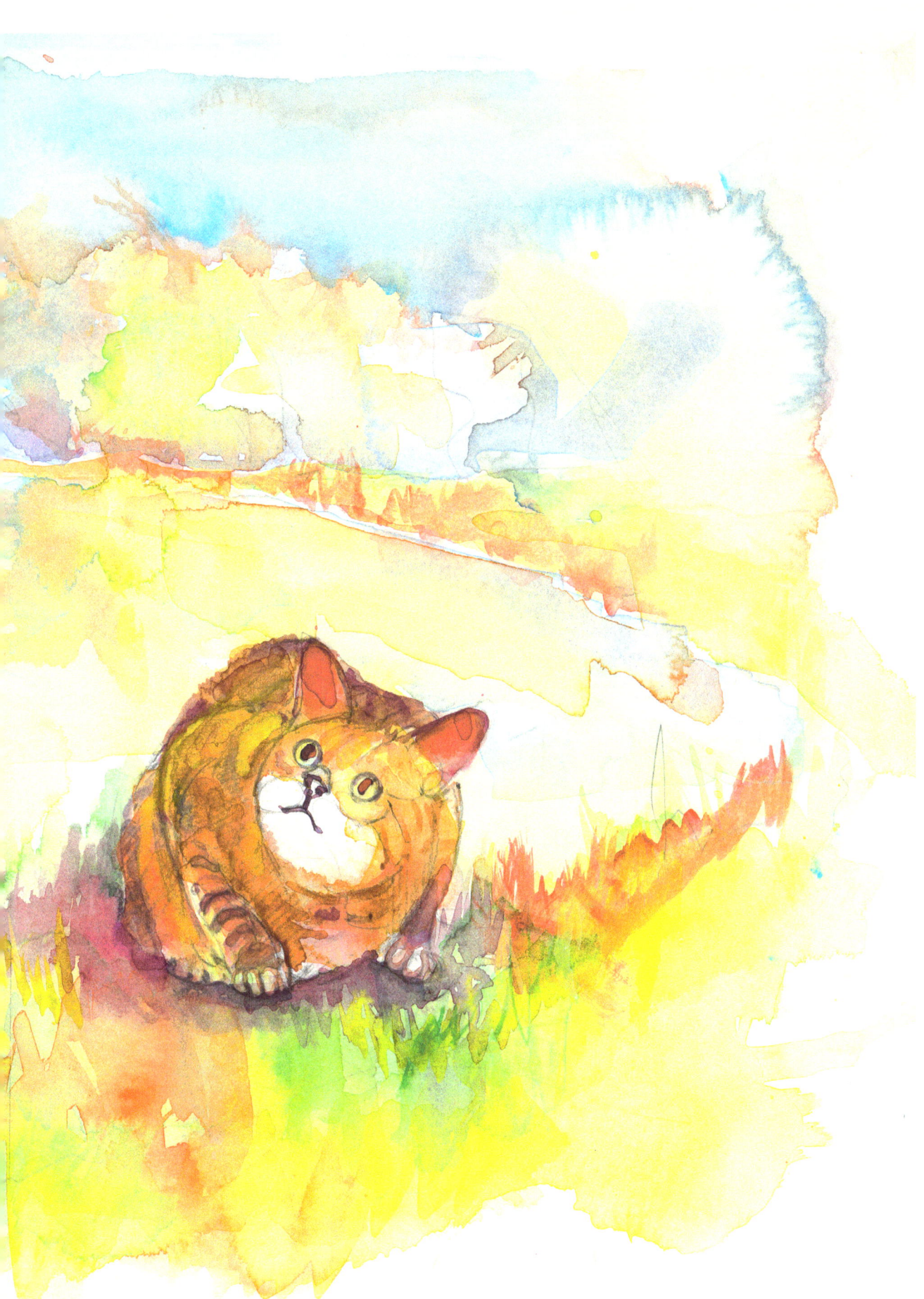

Panda Bear holds its toes...

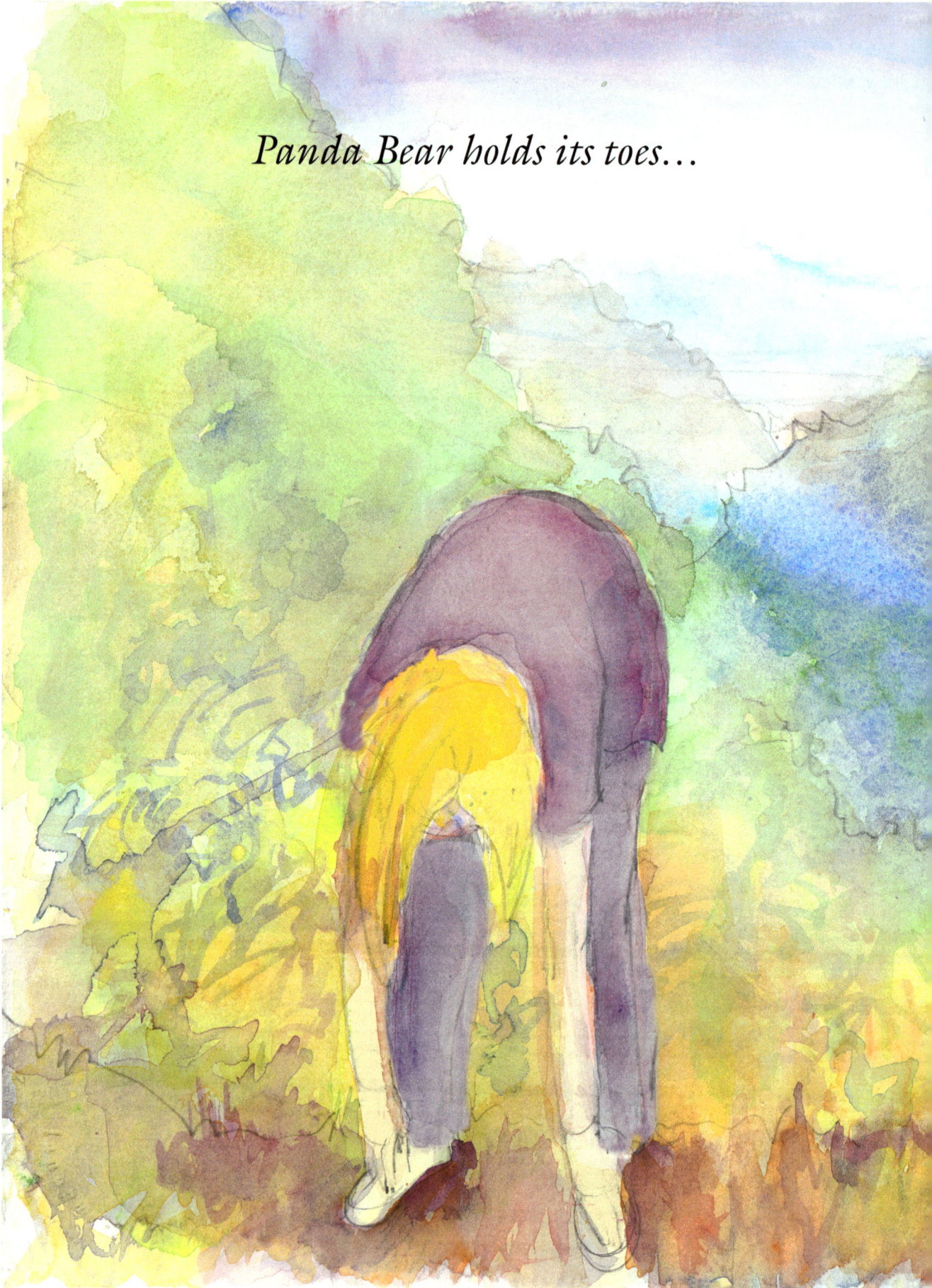

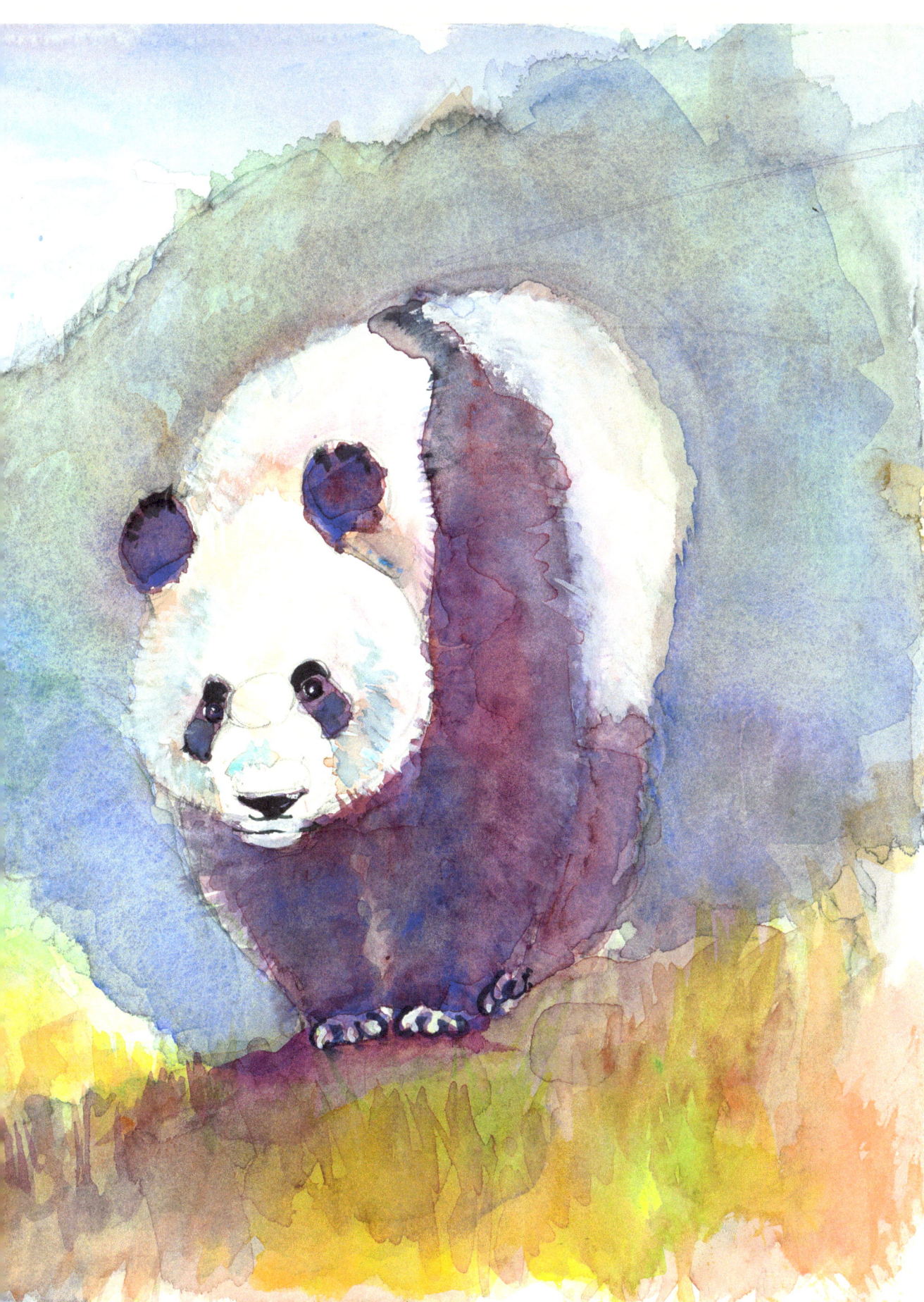

Leaf Green Mantis punches – right then left…

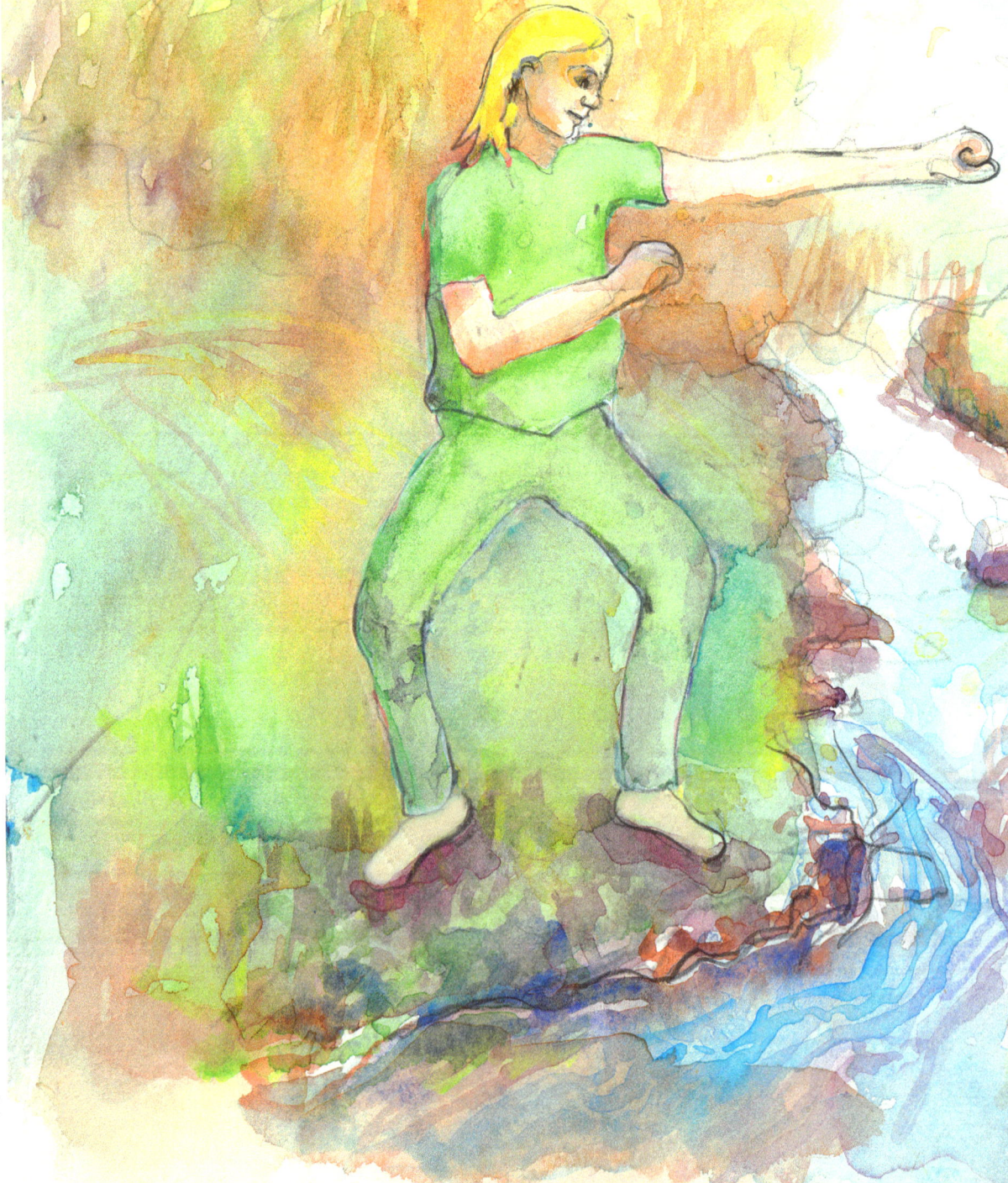

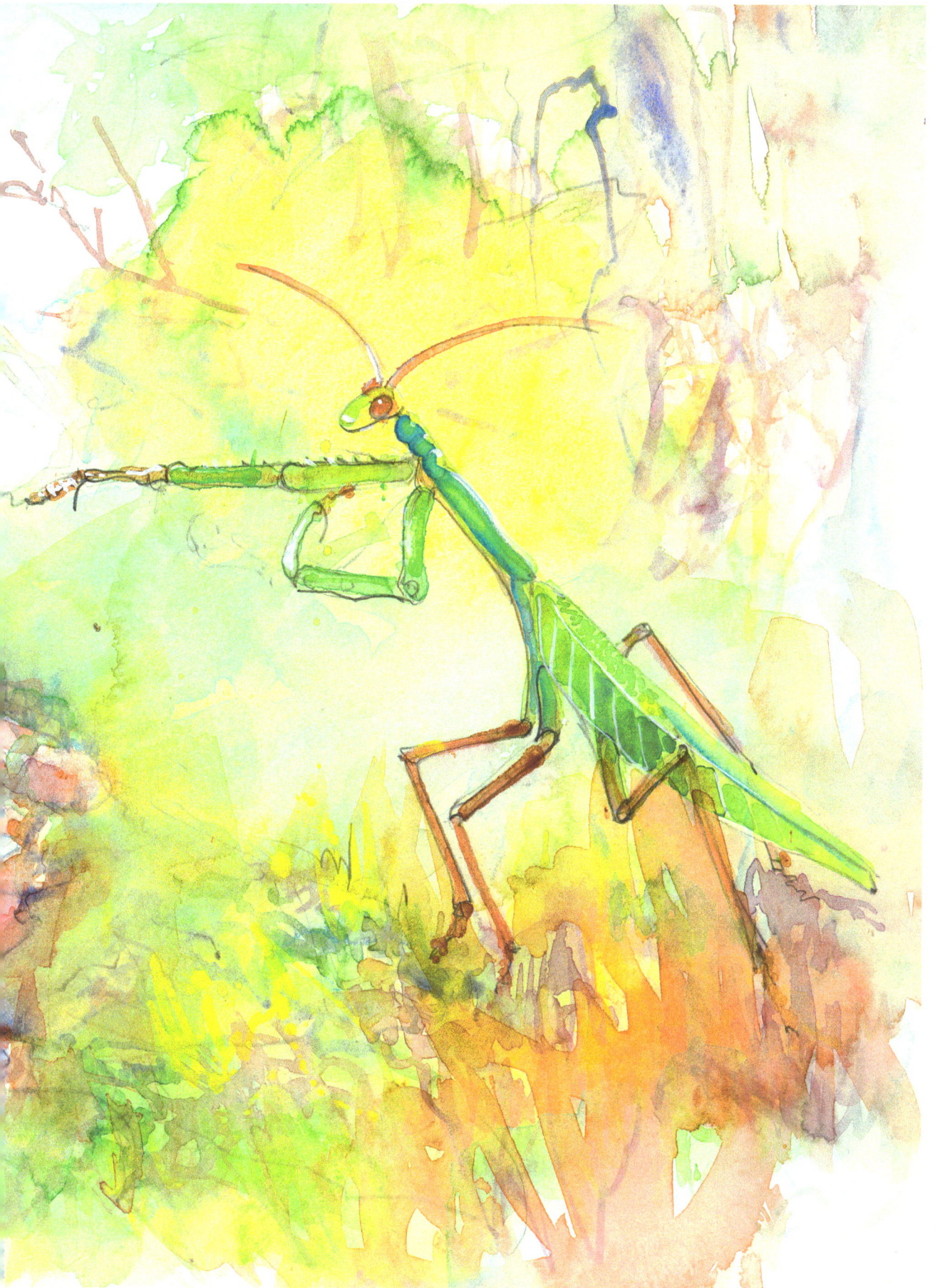

Frisky Rabbit stands on tiptoe...
        then lowers heels with a bump...

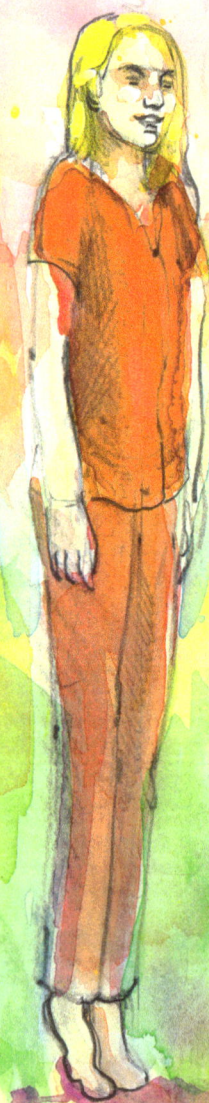

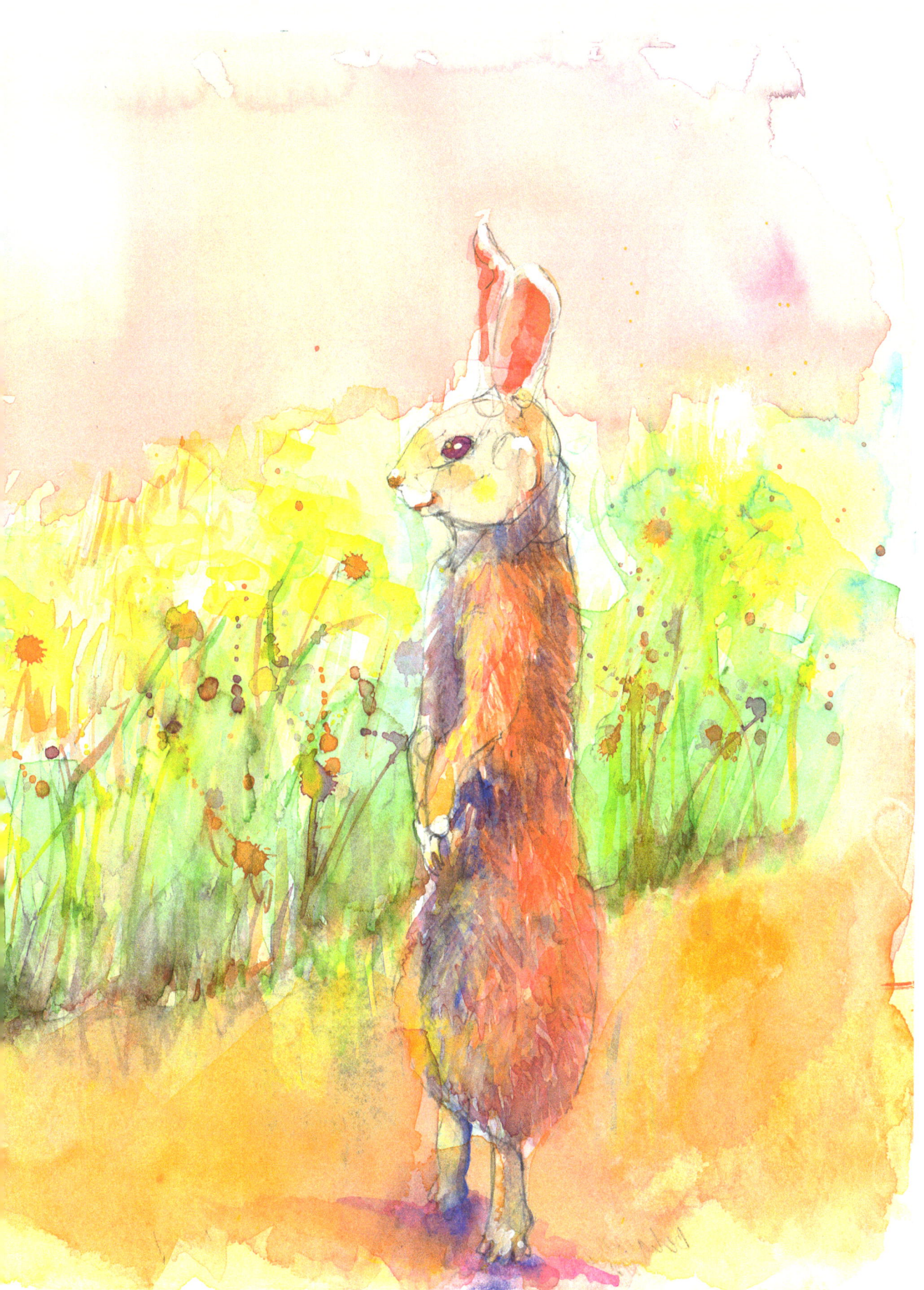

Practicing

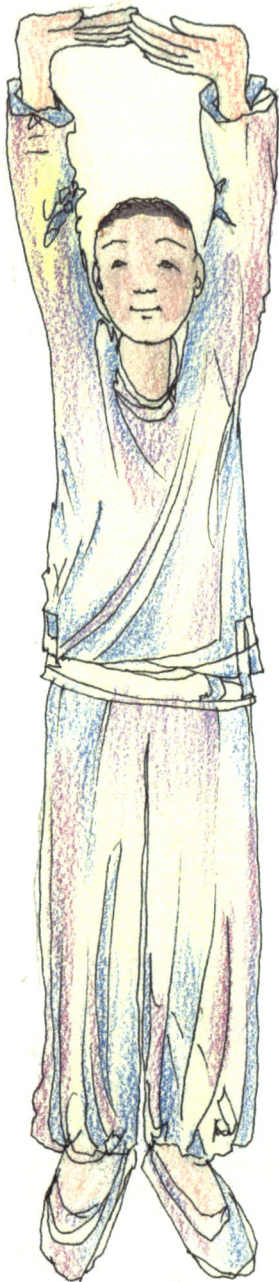

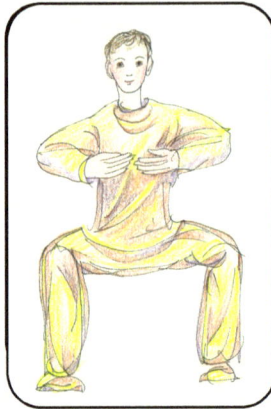

Horse Stance

3 EASY EXERCISES:
Standing, sitting or lying down… try
1. Swinging your arms…
2. Marching in place…
3. Bending your wrists and curling your fingers… Bending your ankles and curling your toes.

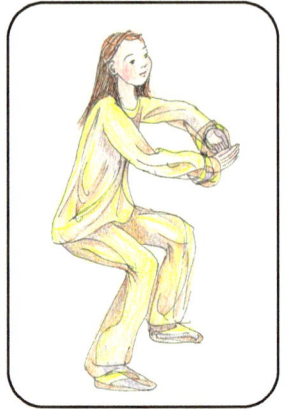

Holding the Ball

Circle arms above head
Fingertips touch
Lean back slightly
Bend side to side

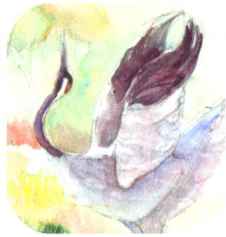

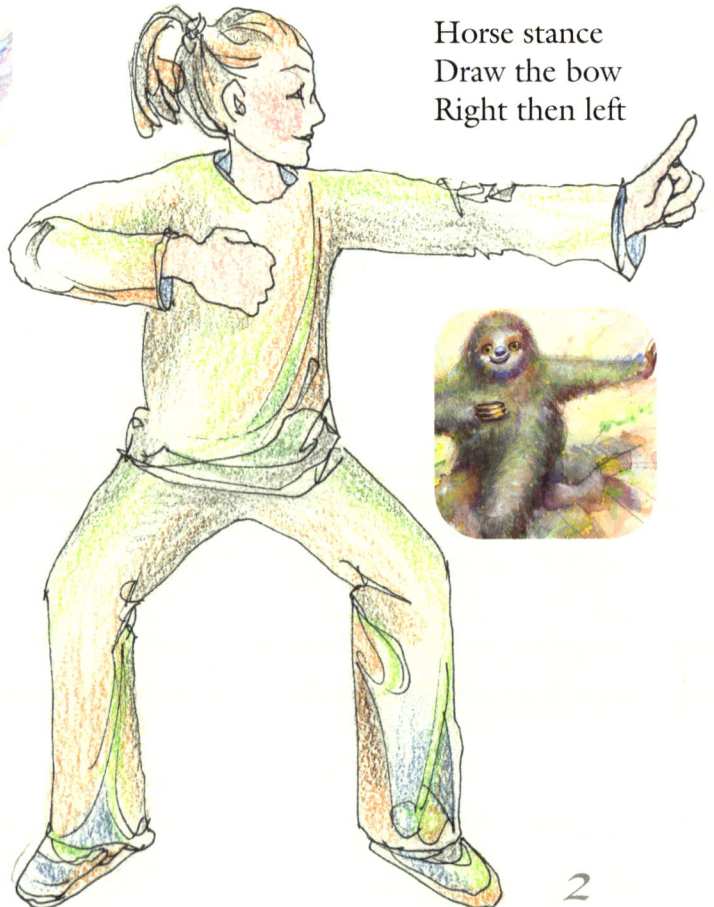

Horse stance
Draw the bow
Right then left

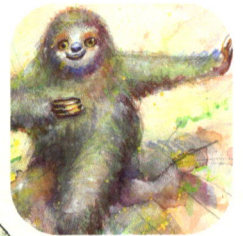

1

2

Sky arm — Earth arm
Push up — push down
Right then left

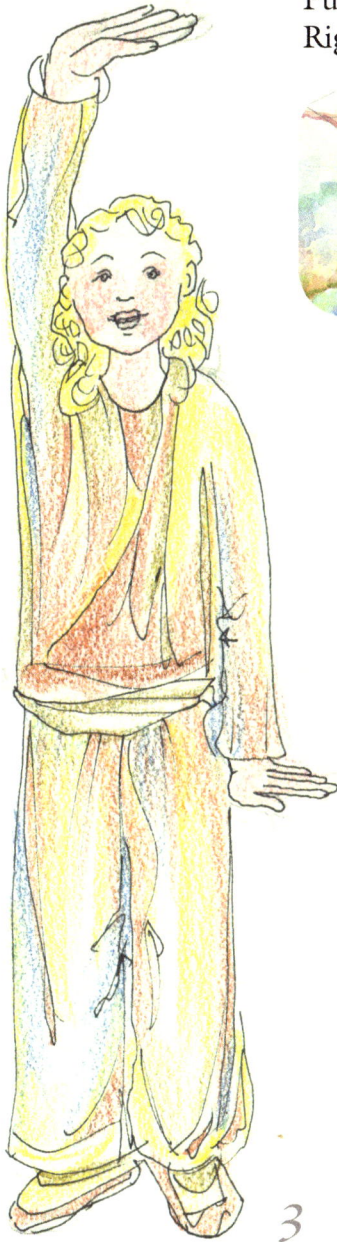

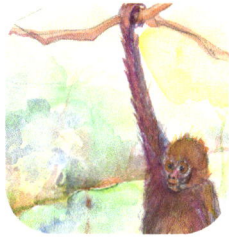

Practicing

3

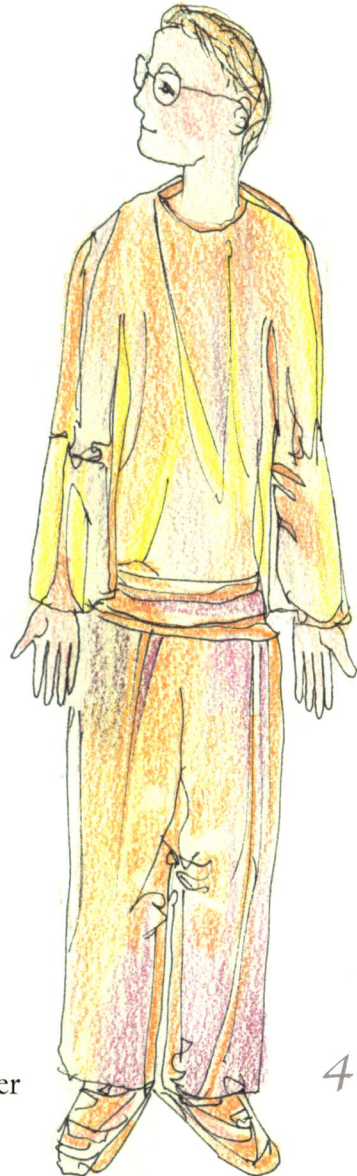

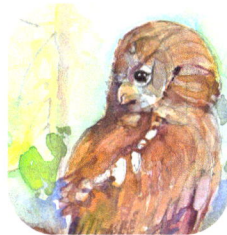

Look back over shoulder
Right then left

4

Practicing

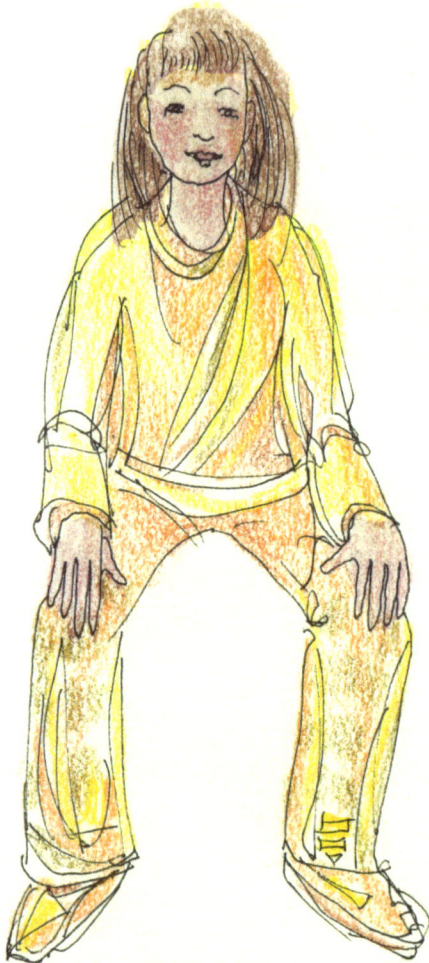

Horse stance
Hands pressed on knees
Bend over right knee
Swing over to left knee
Then back and forth

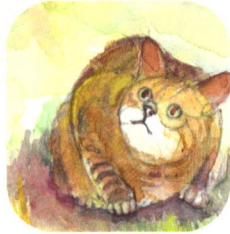

5

Bend back
Then forward
Hold the toes

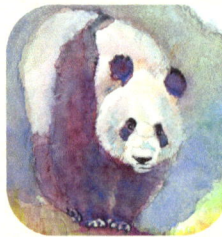

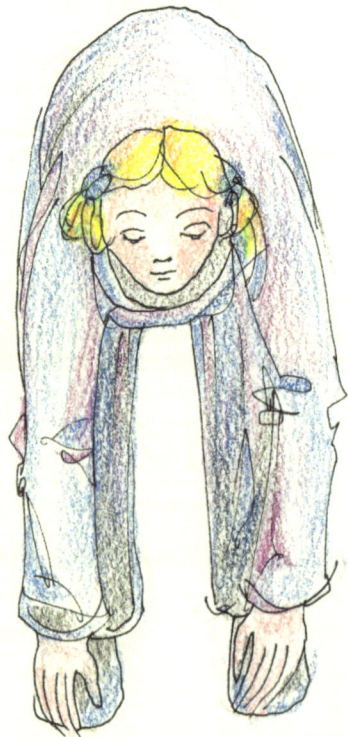

6

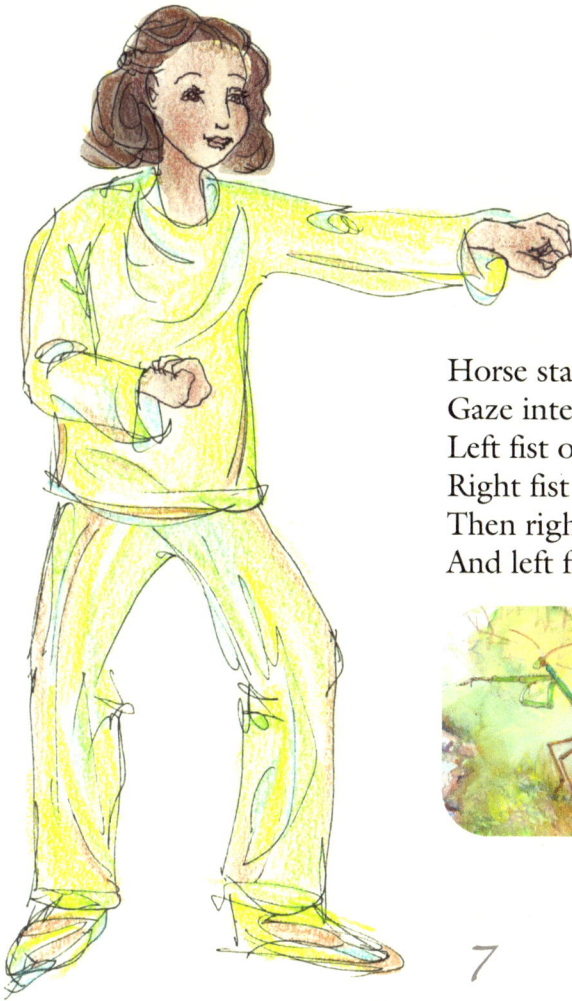

Horse stance
Gaze intently
Left fist out
Right fist back
Then right fist out
And left fist back

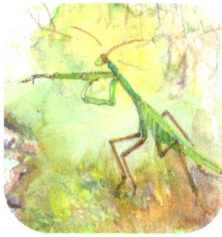

7

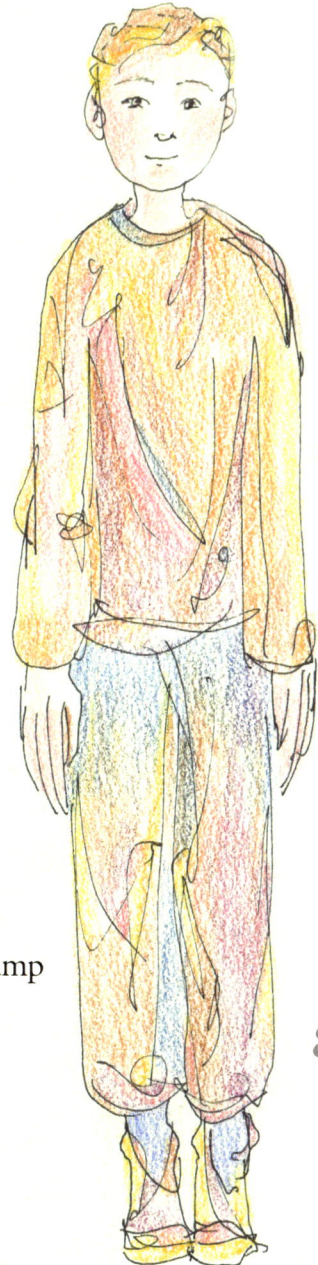

Stand on tiptoe
Three seconds
Lower heels with a bump

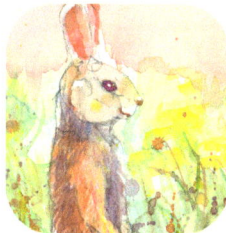

8

If you like to play guessing games... Tell us, please, what are our names?

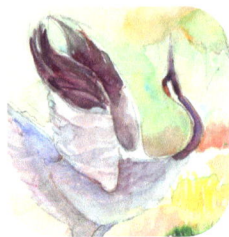

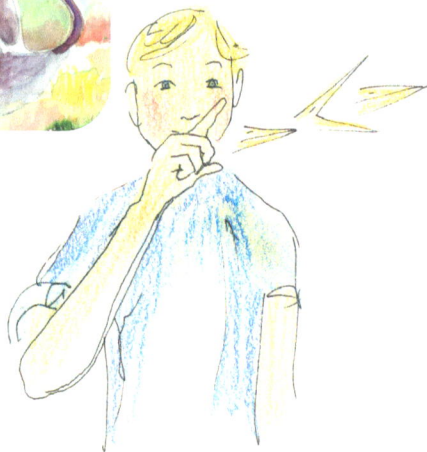

1

Crane

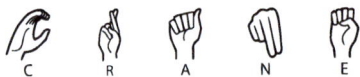

C R A N E

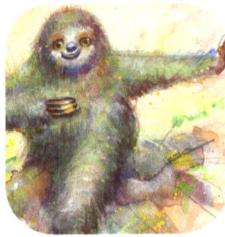

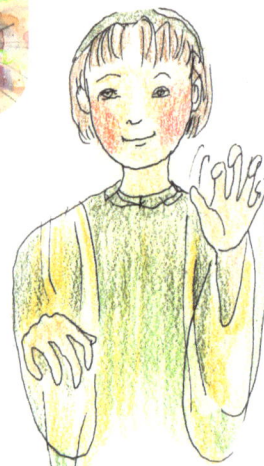

2

Sloth

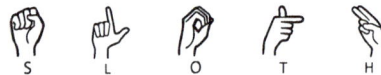

S L O T H

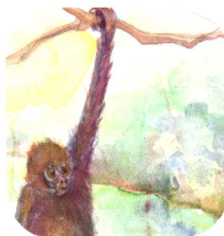

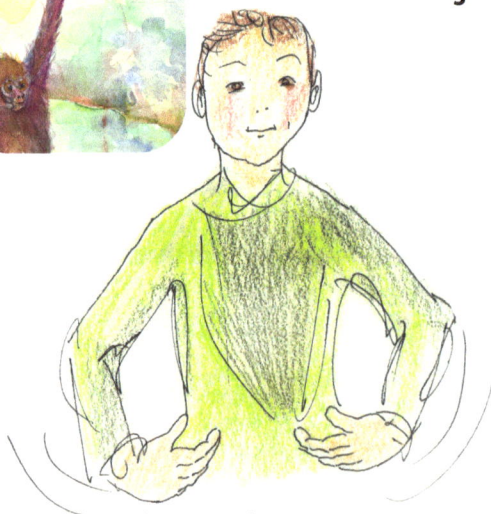

3

Monkey

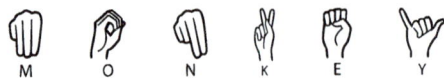

M O N K E Y

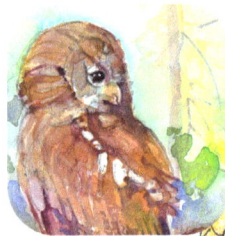

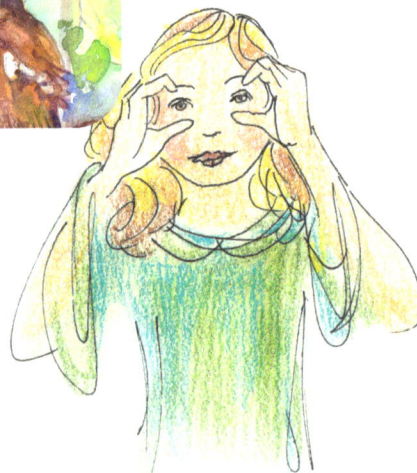

4

Owl

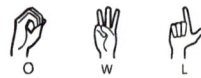

O W L

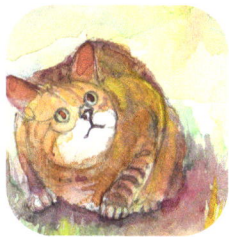

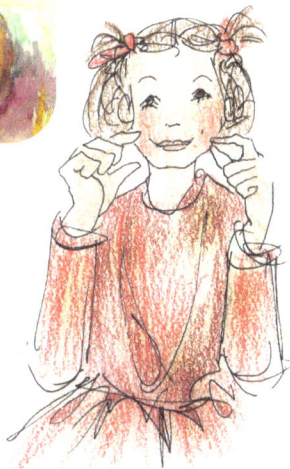

5

Cat

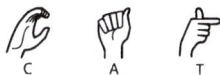

C A T

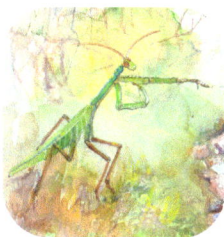

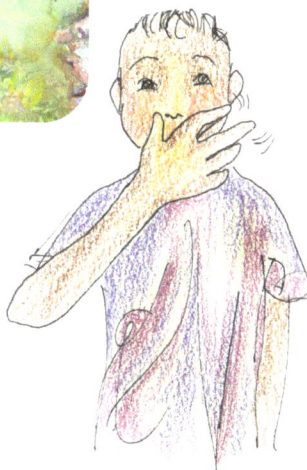

6

Insect

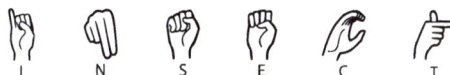

I N S E C T

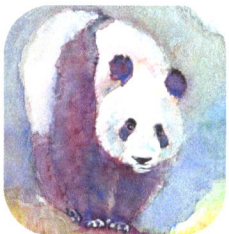

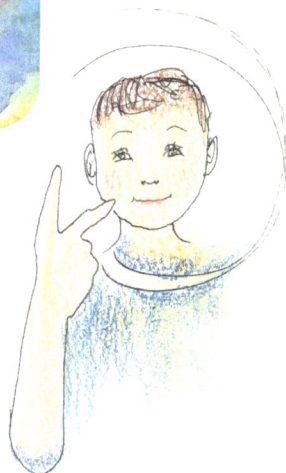

7

Panda

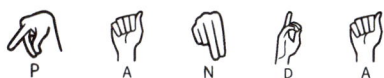

P A N D A

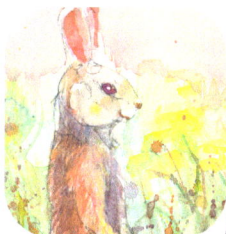

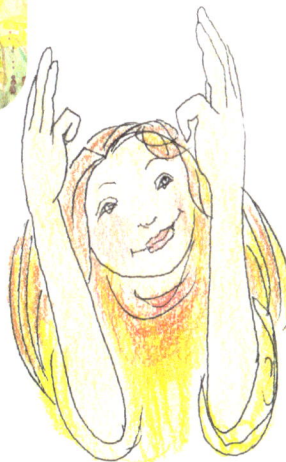

8

Rabbit

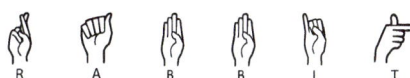

R A B B I T

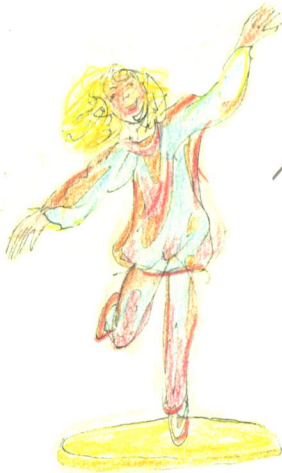

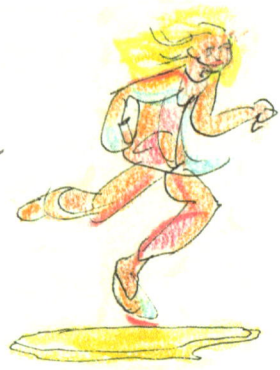

Will you, won't you,

will you, won't you,

will you join the dance?

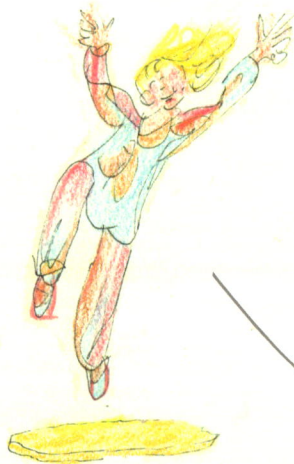

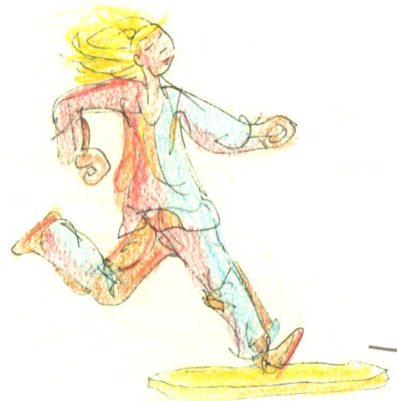

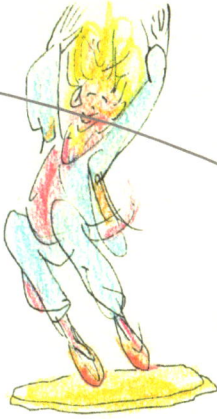

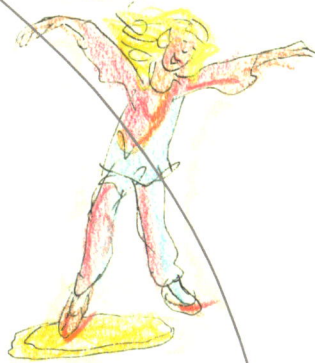

Will you, won't you,

will you, won't you,

won't you join the dance?

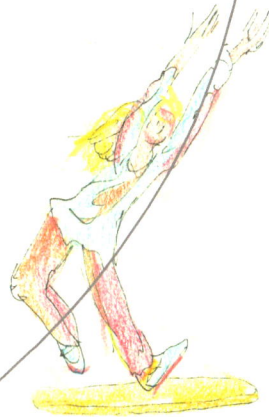

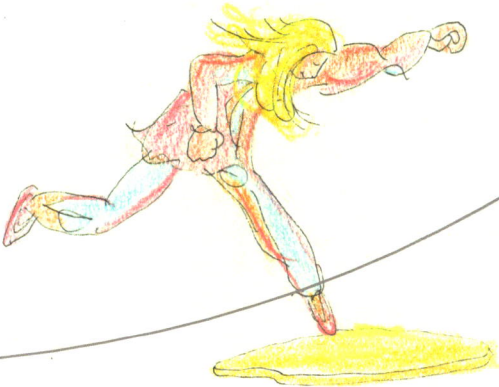

I

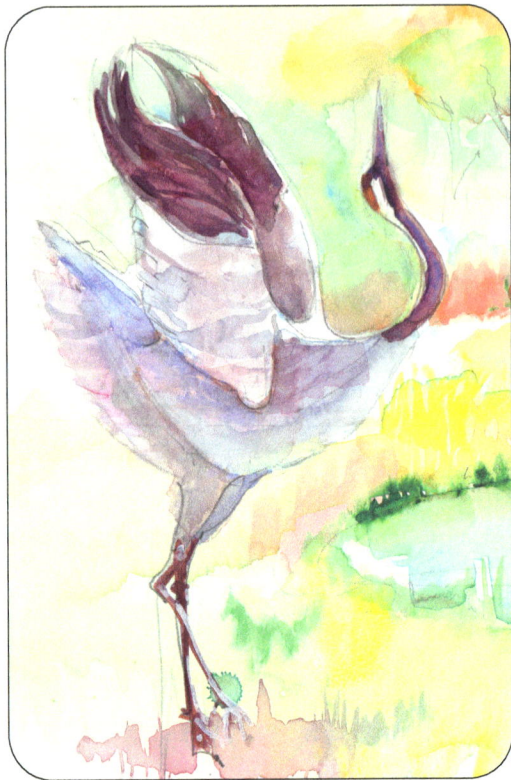

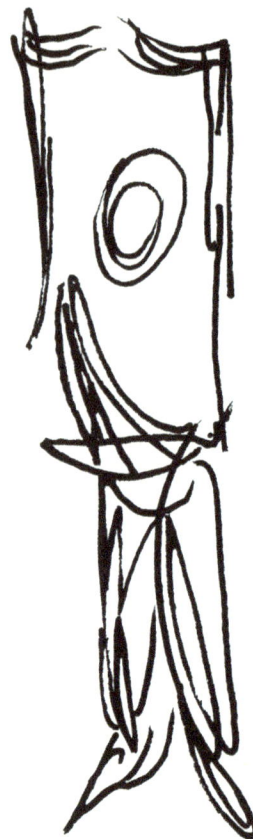

II

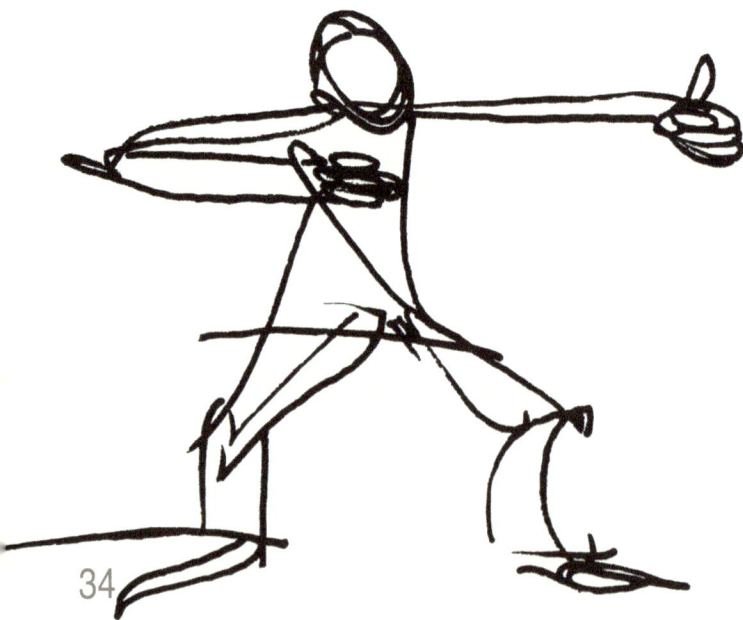

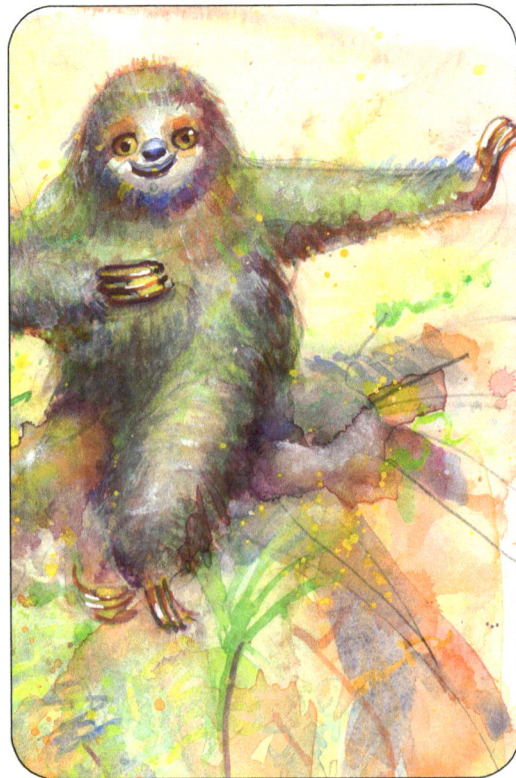

34

III

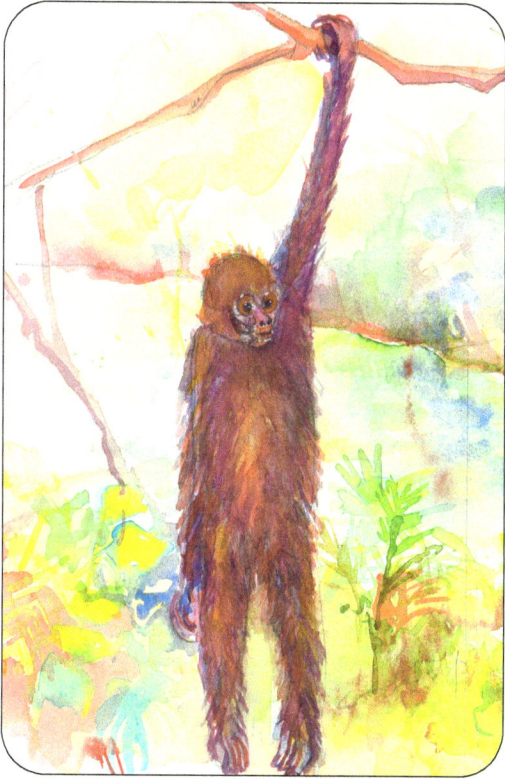

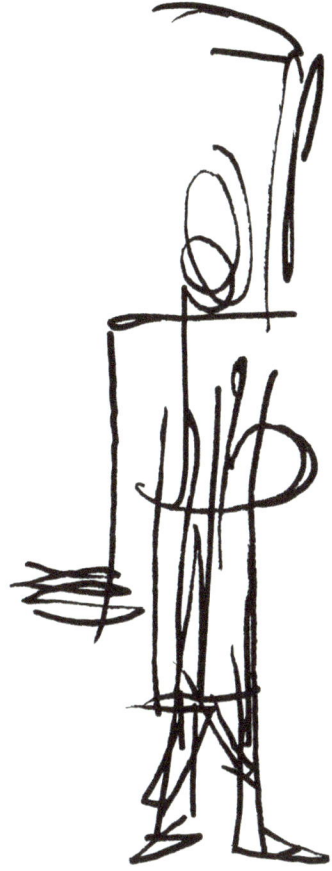

IV

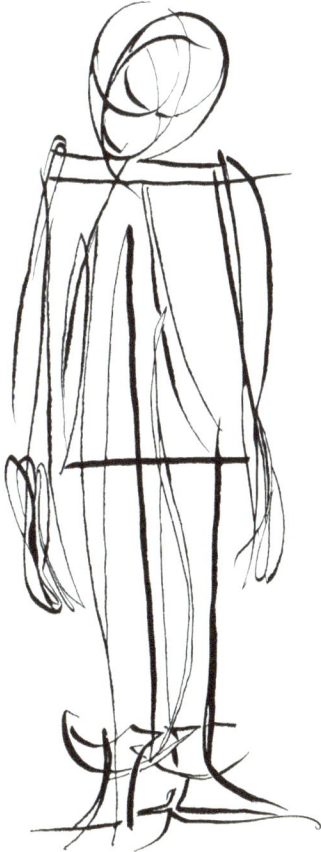

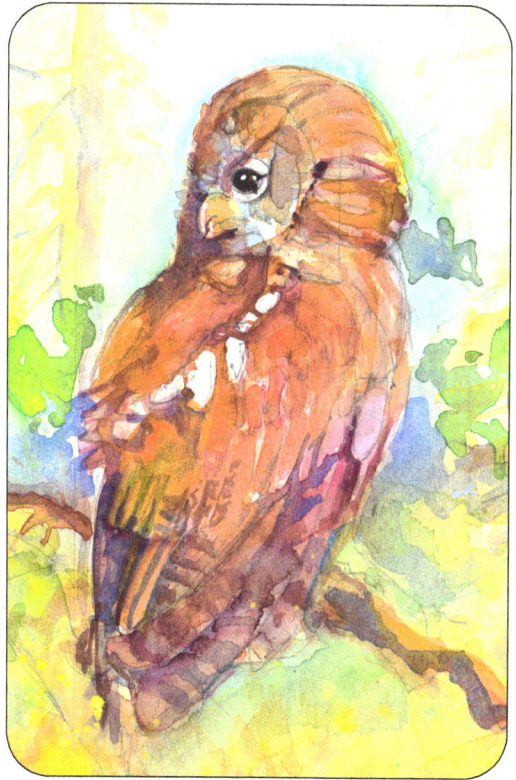

35

V

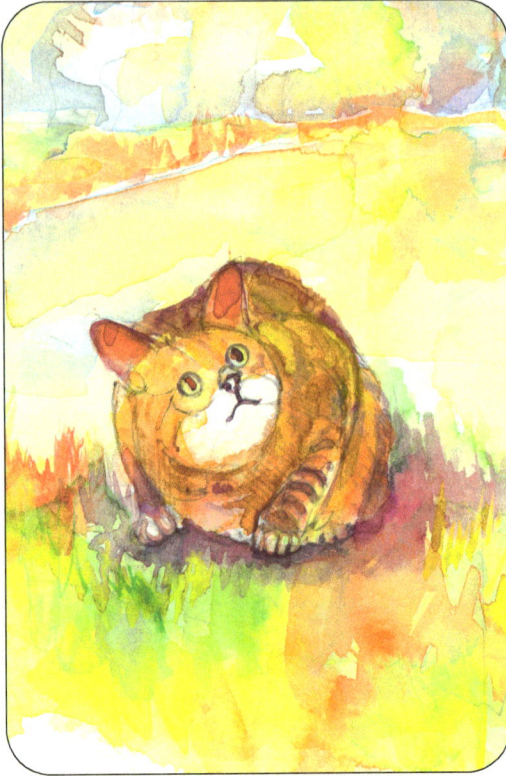

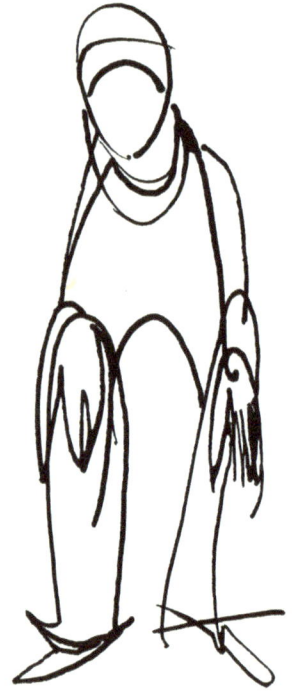

VI

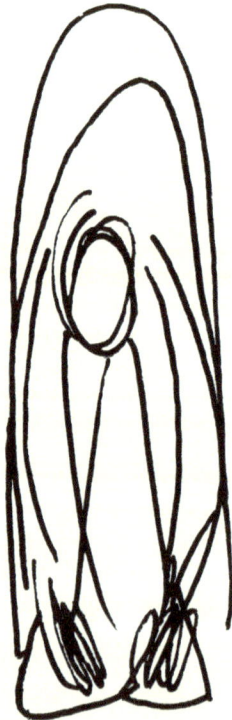

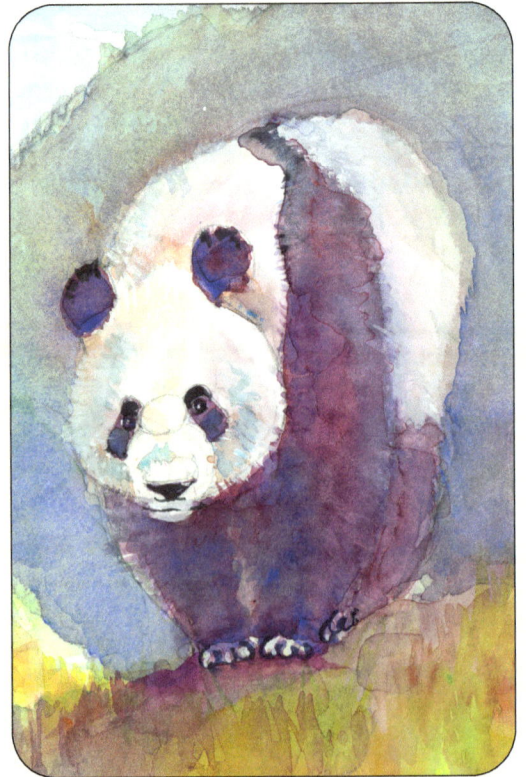

VII

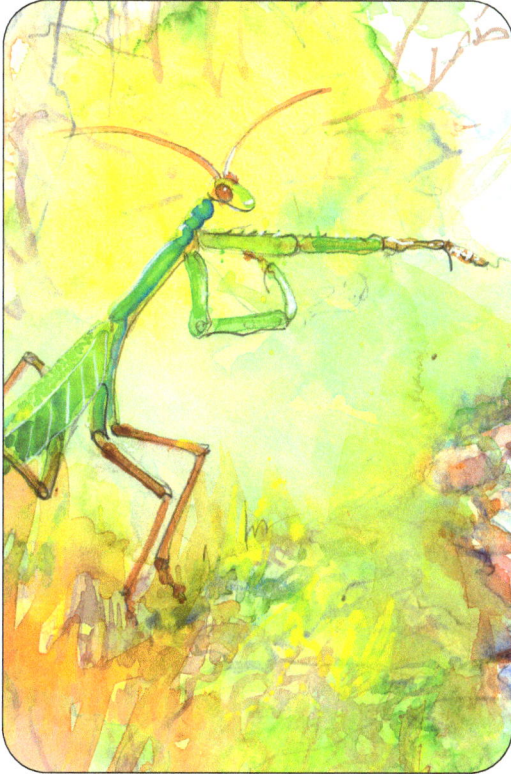

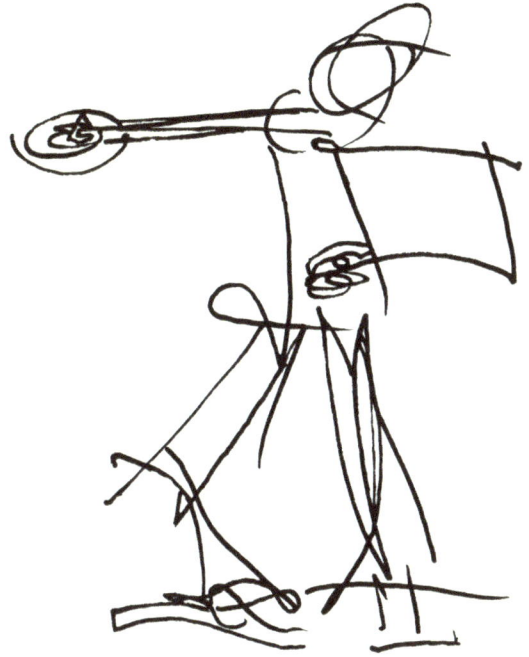

VIII

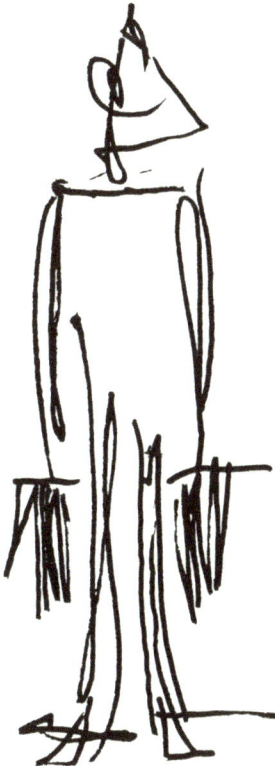

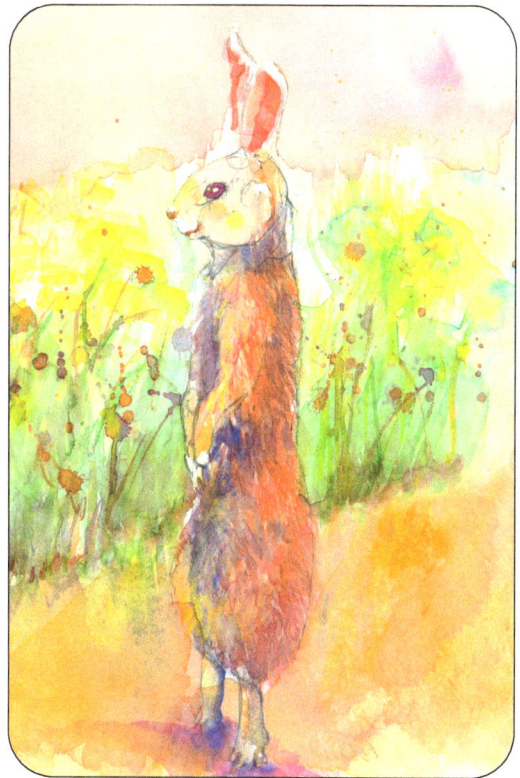

prrractice

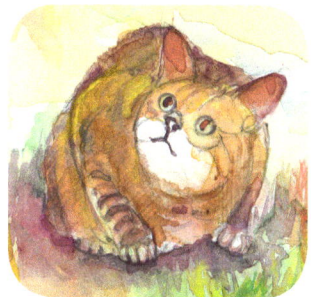

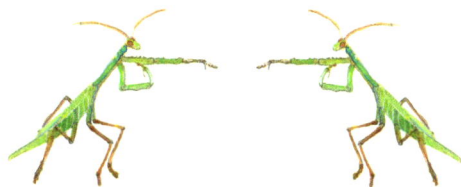

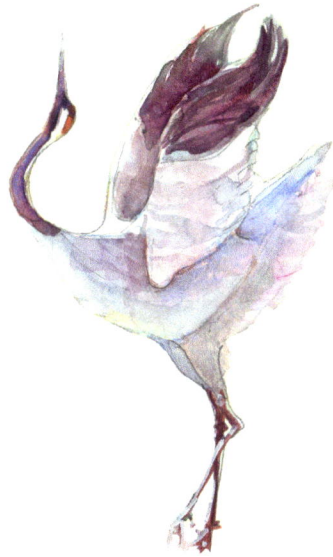

www.ingramcontent.com/pod-product-compliance
Lightning Source LLC
Chambersburg PA
CBHW042100040426
42448CB00002B/87